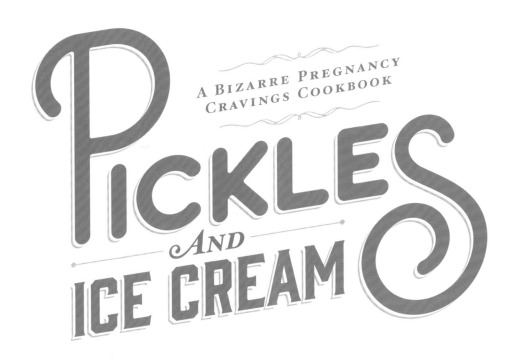

PICKLES AND ICE CREAM

A Bizarre Pregnancy Cravings Cookbook

VICKY JACOB-EBBINGHAUS
& JUAREZ RODRIGUES

ROBINSON

ROBINSON

First published in the US in 2017 by Running Press, an imprint of Perseus Books, LLC

First published in Great Britain in 2017 by Robinson

1 2 3 4 5 6 7 8 9 10

A CIP catalogue record for this book is available from the British Library.

ISBN: 978-1-47213-942-9

The third party trademarks used in this book are the property of their respective owners, including but not limited to the owners of M&M's®, Mars®, Oreo®, and Skittles®. The owners of these trademarks have not endorsed, authorized, or sponsored this book.

Cover and interior design by Juarez Rodrigues and Jason Kayser
Edited by Jennifer Kasius
Typography: Gotham and Mercury

Printed and bound in China

Papers used by Robinson are from well-managed forests and other responsible sources.

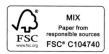

Robinson
An imprint of
Little, Brown Book Group
Carmelite House
50 Victoria Embankment
London EC4Y 0DZ

An Hachette UK Company
www.hachette.co.uk

www.littlebrown.co.uk

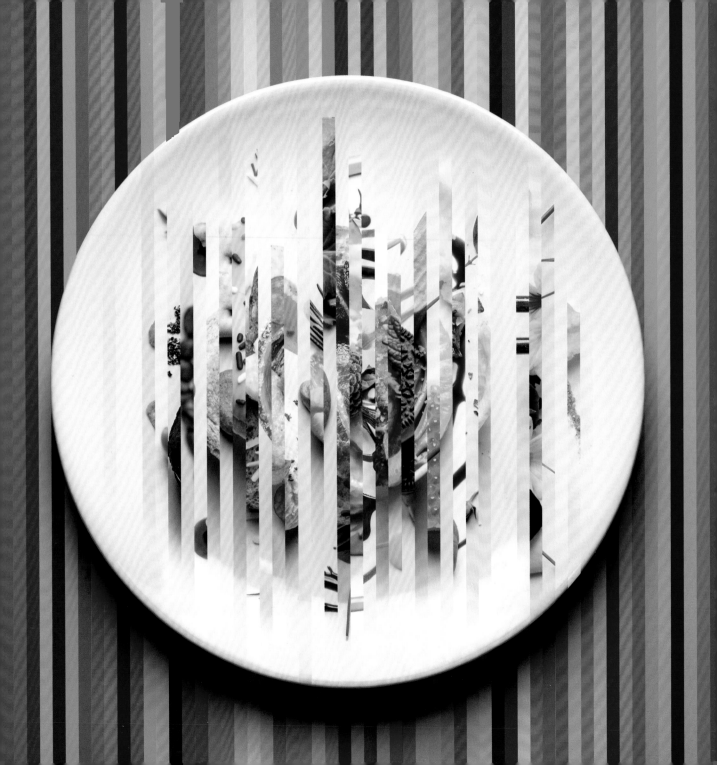

CONTENTS

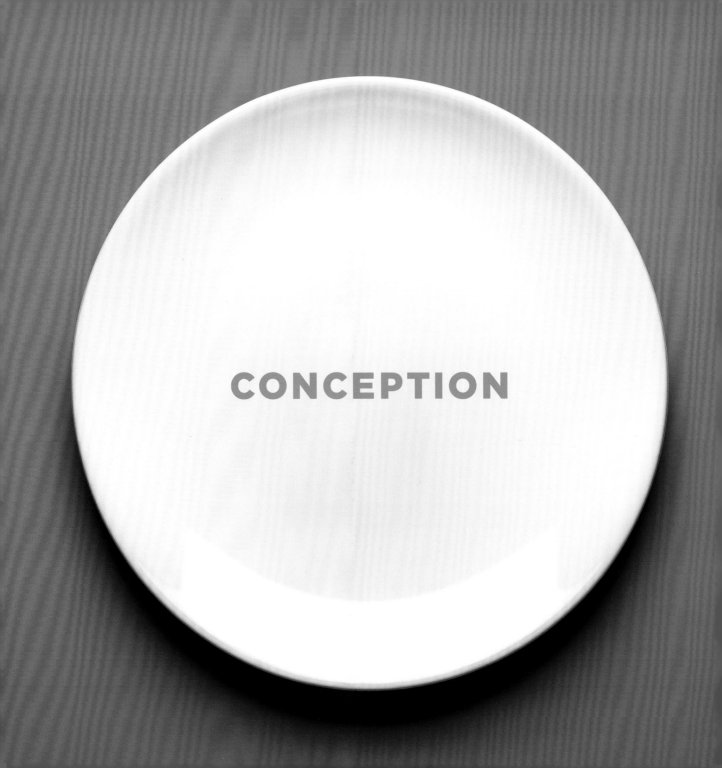

CONCEPTION

THIS BOOK WAS CONCEIVED RIGHT AFTER A CONFESSION OF LOVE WAS MADE. IT WAS ONE OF THOSE FORBIDDEN TYPES OF LOVE THAT SOCIETY WOULD SAY WAS NEVER MEANT TO BE. THE LOVE BETWEEN A WOMAN . . . AND TOOTHPASTE WITH COOKIES.

When our friend admitted to eating this strange combo, we would have thought her mad if it hadn't been for one thing—something that instantly downgraded her to just "mildly eccentric" on the crazy scale. She was pregnant. And as we all know, having a miniature human growing inside of you can really mess with how your tongue and brain work. For our friend regular Oreos suddenly became like Charlie Chaplin without his moustache. The Internet without cats. A Michael Bay movie without explosions. Just . . . missing something. Once she had given birth, however, the craving disappeared. The toothpaste moved from the kitchen back to the bathroom and was dutifully spat out twice a day without the slightest urge to swallow.

This sudden transition from the disgusting to the delicious and back again fascinated us. We knew the classic stories of husbands and partners making midnight runs for some bizarre item. Or women whipping up ingredient combinations that only a mother-to-be could love. And we began to wonder what strange concoctions pregnant women were creating. Then and there, we decided to make the world's first crazy pregnancy cravings recipe book. We would collect all the pregnancy cravings we could find, the weirder, the better. And we would somehow find a way to make them look as delicious as they tasted to the women who craved them.

What followed next was over a year of research. We spoke to every single person we knew who had ever made use of their uterus. Beginning with family, friends, and acquaintances and then graduating onto strangers and random passersby. We devoured all the literature we could on the subject, engaged on forums and social media, set up questionnaires, and trawled through comment sections. And although we stopped short of loitering in maternity wards, it was a close call.

During our research we estimate we looked at around 50,000 pregnancy cravings from all over the world. We learned that some women developed strong food aversions: things that used to make their mouths water suddenly made their stomachs heave. Others became obsessed with one or two foods and created maniacally monotonous breakfast, lunch, and dinner menus for themselves. Still others craved very strange items or unusual combinations. And some craved nothing at all.

During this time, we didn't just discover amazing cravings, we met some amazing people, too. And although almost everyone we spoke to was happy to share their experiences with us, sadly a lot of women had been ashamed of their cravings when they had them. This made us even more determined to continue with the project. We wanted women to know that when it came to weird cravings, they most certainly weren't alone. And no matter how bizarre their eating habits were, there was a good chance someone had craved something weirder.

MAKING OUR BABY

Once we had our list of the best, worst, and most random pregnancy cravings, we set to work. But shopping for the recipes came with its own problems. It's one thing to go to the checkout with arms full of pickle jars or enough toothpaste for a lifetime of sparkling smiles. It's another thing entirely to hang around a busy playground waiting for the right moment to surreptitiously put a few handfuls of sand into a plastic bag. Or walk around your neighborhood with a hammer in your backpack, looking for a condemned building to "harvest" some cement walls for a recipe. Being based in Germany at the time of writing, some items were almost impossible to find. What do you do when you have a recipe for "Pickled Pig's Foot with Cornflakes and Milk," but pickled pig's feet aren't sold in Germany? As it turns out, you go to a butcher, get an entire pig's lower leg and then cook and pickle it yourself. Not a job for the squeamish. Or those with an aversion to feet. Pity that we fell into both those categories. And where do you even start looking for lamb's eyes? This little nightmare of a craving was from a vegetarian whose meat cravings got out of hand while walking through a market in Morocco.

Even after practicing our very best "I am not a creepy weirdo" voices (is it more disturbing to ask for lamb's eyes with or without a smile?), the conversation in every butcher shop and restaurant still inevitably went like this:

Us: "Hi, I was wondering if you have any lamb's eyes?"

"Lamb's eyes?"

"Yes . . . raw or cooked is fine."

". . ."

(We muster the least sinister smile possible)

"Ok, thank you."

(Leave store making a mental note to never set foot in there again)

Eventually we ended up at a small Turkish restaurant.

Here the conversation started off as usual before taking a slight different turn.

"**Hi, I was wondering if you have any lamb's eyes?**"

"**Lamb's eyes?**"

"**Yes . . . raw or cooked is fine.**"

"**Just the eyes? You don't want the whole head? We normally just sell the whole head.**"

Now it was our turn to pause. First for a quick check that the proprietor wasn't joking—his expression seemed to suggest he wasn't. And also to mentally run through the implications of getting a whole head instead of just the eyes. Somehow the thought of a skinned lamb's head glaring at us every time we opened the fridge was rather terrifying. Interpreting the pause as indecision, he disappeared into the back and returned a few moments later with five roasted lamb's heads on a tray. Perhaps he felt a short introduction would help us feel more comfortable as he immediately picked up one of the lamb's heads and began moving the jaw while saying "**Hellooo!**" in a high-pitched voice—obviously his best impression of what a lamb might sound like if it could talk . . . and somehow found itself detached from its body and having an idle conversation in a restaurant.

He grinned. The decapitated lamb grinned ghoulishly. Silence stretched out.

"**Hellooo!**" it repeated.

It was clearly waiting for a response.

"**Hello,**" we mumbled back sheepishly—apt, considering the circumstances.

Once again there was a moment of silence. We were used to awkward conversations but one with a lamb's head was a whole new experience. "How are you?" felt like a strange question considering that the lamb was very obviously not fine at all. And it felt all kinds of wrong to address the lamb directly when asking for its eyes, so we aimed our next question back at the lamb ventriloquist.

"**Could we just get the eyes?**"

He stared at us. The lamb stared at us. We avoided eye contact.

Thankfully he put the head down.

"**To eat here or take away?**"

"**To take away please. It's for a photography project.**"

He took this in his stride and simply nodded like people wanting to photograph lamb's eyes was a completely normal thing to do. Or maybe he just thought we were trying to pull the equivalent of unnecessarily blurting out to a store clerk "I'm just buying these condoms for a friend! They aren't for me!"

"**You want them all?**"

Another unexpected turn of events. We thought we would be lucky to get two. Now we had the option of ten.

"**Sure!**"

With that, he grabbed a spoon and began to cheerfully pop the eyes out of the skulls and put them in a Styrofoam takeaway box.

As one of the more surreal chapters of our lives came to a close, we left the restaurant with our box of lambs' eyes, too afraid to look back in case we heard that high-pitched voice and saw the now eyeless lamb's skull uttering a last **"Good-byyyye!"**

* * *

The next challenge for us was creating the recipes. Being the consummate professionals we were, we set up a makeshift photo studio in the bedroom by balancing a tripod on an Ikea chest over a small dining room table. With a good few years of cooking and eating under our belts, we were filled with the overconfidence we needed to believe this would be easy. Our first attempts at both re-creating recipes and food styling can be summarized by an endless loop of this conversation:

"Maybe we should just add a little more of this."

"OK."

"Damn it. That was too much, wasn't it?"

"Yes."

"All right. Let's start again."

Luckily, thanks to the prestigious School of Trial and Error and the esteemed Academy of the Internet, we eventually started to make some headway.

We were also stupidly committed to tasting every single recipe. The world needed to know what these dishes were like to an objective, nonpregnant palate. And we felt obligated to provide those palates. Surprisingly, the first few dishes were really good. As brave, new explorers in the world of pregnancy cravings, we had been expecting all manner of horrors. But the Toothpaste Oreos just tasted like minty Oreos. The Bacon Mars Bar Burger was delicious. We were beginning to think that these crazy pregnancy cravings might just be the genius kind of crazy.

Right up until we were sitting on either side of a plate of brightly colored soaps.

"Try it."

"No, you try it first."

"No, YOU try it!"

A long staring contest ensued. Tension was in the air. That song from *The Good, the Bad and the Ugly* was playing softly in the background.

"Ok, we try it together."

We both tried it. All illusions of genius died instantly.

It took many, many dirty words, many, many mouth rinses, and a good few Bacon Mars Bar Burgers before we could bring ourselves to continue with the project. But continue we did. And survive we did.

We started the cookbook as the online blog "Eating for Two Cookbook." Two weeks later, much to our shock and delight, the recipes went viral, shocking and delighting people all over the world.

A WORD ABOUT PICA

We discovered a lot of things when making this book. Like that an open can of sauerkraut can really stink up your fridge. And it's difficult to get chocolate to stick to shrimp. But one of the most surprising things was that a lot of pregnant women crave nonfood items. Things like bricks, dirt, sponges, nail polish, or soap. This is a condition called *pica* and can sometimes be related to a zinc or iron deficiency. Although one of us does own a white coat, neither of us is a real doctor. And a genuine, qualified doctor is someone you should most definitely seek out if you are craving anything along these lines.

We spent a lot of time stroking our beards (one real, one imaginary) trying to decide whether we should include these pica cravings in the book. On the one hand, we don't want anyone to think that we in any way support eating things that might be dangerous for a mother or baby. On the other hand, this is a book about what real pregnant women crave and eat. Not what they *should* eat. In the end we included them because we have faith in humanity's ability to avoid things clearly labeled as "do not eat." Please, don't destroy that faith!

THE CRAVING RATING SCALE

It was while we were treating our taste buds to a variety of delights and traumas that we set up our star rating scale. Each and every recipe was tasted and rated on this highly scientific review system based on mood and personal taste. It is deciphered below for your reference.

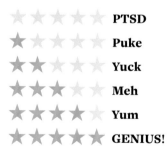

☆ ☆ ☆ ☆ ☆ **PTSD**
★ ☆ ☆ ☆ ☆ **Puke**
★ ★ ☆ ☆ ☆ **Yuck**
★ ★ ★ ☆ ☆ **Meh**
★ ★ ★ ★ ☆ **Yum**
★ ★ ★ ★ ★ **GENIUS!**

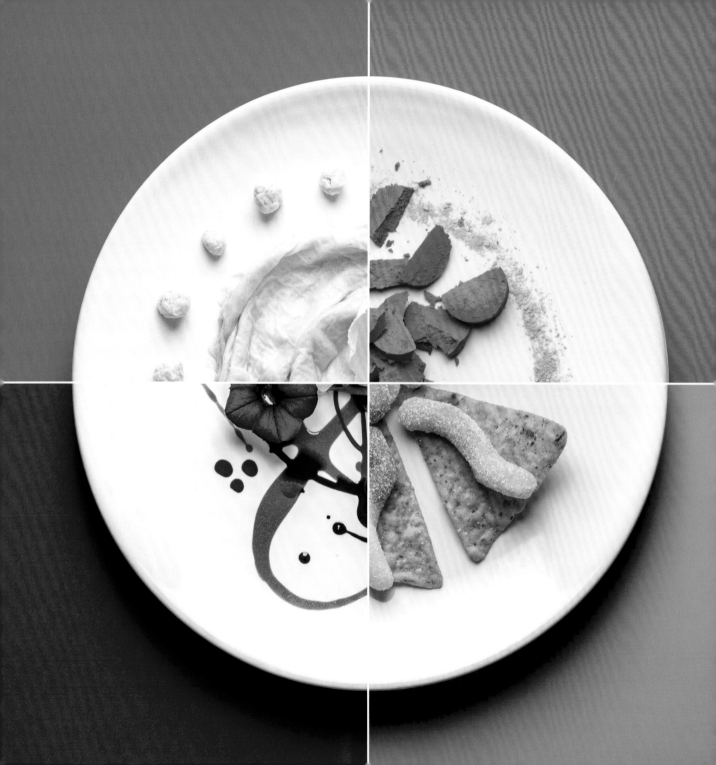

STARTERS

It begins. The first cravings hit. As do the first waves of nausea. Either of which may be the tip-off that you are no longer alone—even when you are by yourself. Which is officially the creepiest way to describe pregnancy.

In this chapter, we have some light snacks, soups, finger food, and appetizers made from the finest ingredients that you can pick at your local supermarket . . . or hardware store. Get ready to drool. And maybe puke a little.

PINEAPPLE AND TROUT CAVIAR CRACKERS

Ludmilla, Moscow, Russia

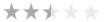

The juice from the pineapple along with the caviar makes it a bit slimy, but hey, giving birth and having babies is a great way to get over squeamishness.

INGREDIENTS

3 large slices of pineapple

2 teaspoons trout caviar

METHOD

Trim the slices of pineapple into equal rectangles.

Add a dollop of caviar to each one—about ⅔ teaspoon per pineapple cracker.

SERVES 1

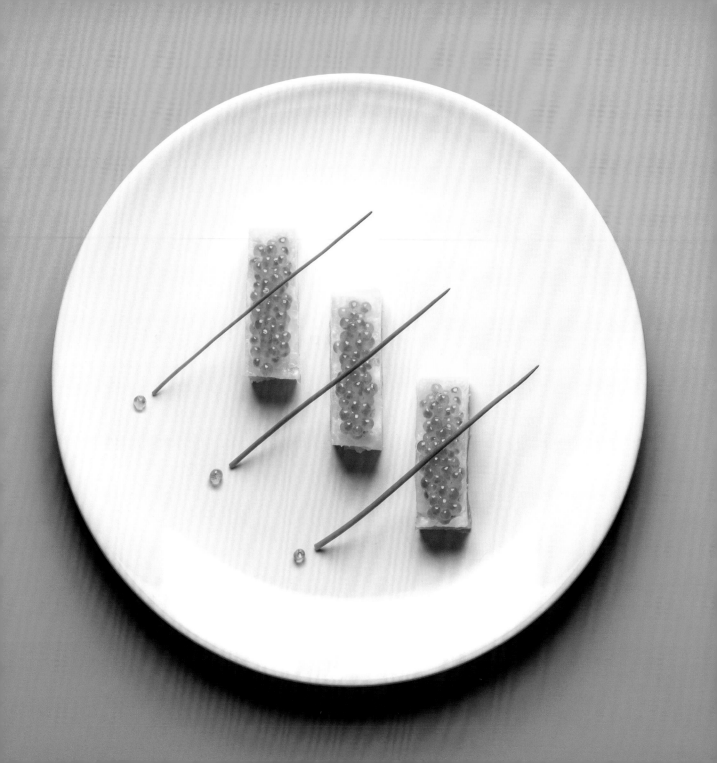

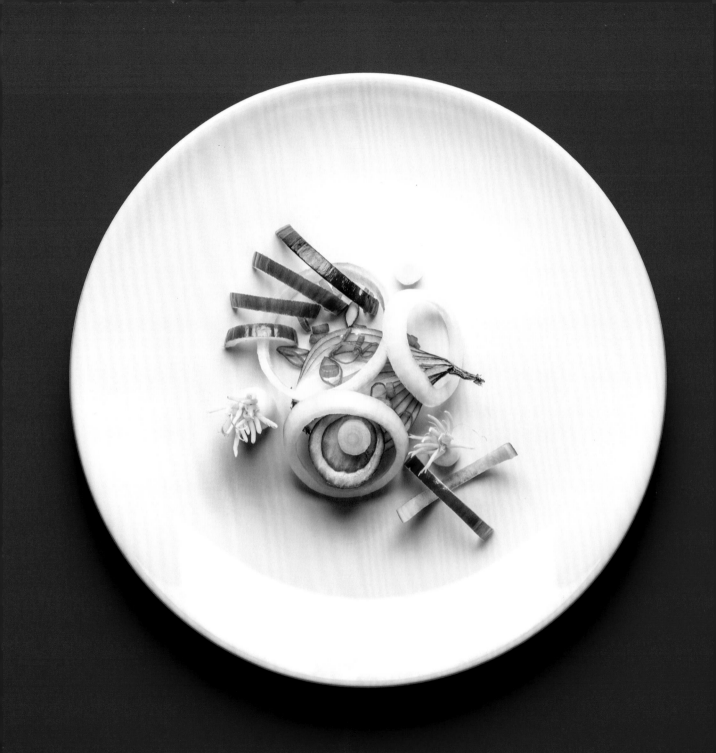

RAW ONIONS

Jessica, Vancouver, Washington, USA

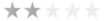

Onion ... the vegetable that goes with anything, but never nothing.

INGREDIENTS

*½ onion, red, white, or mixed
according to preference*

1 spring onion, for garnish

METHOD

Slice the onions into rings and bite-size pieces.

Arrange the rings and pieces on a plate. Consider making a design like the Olympic rings, an animal, or an abstract artwork.

Slice up the spring onion and sprinkle over the plate.

If all the slicing takes up too much time, simply peel the onion and take a bite.

SERVES 1

RAW
ONIONS

JESSICA, VANCOUVER, WASHINGTON, USA

I WAS PREGNANT WITH MY OLDEST IN 2004 AND CRAVED ONIONS LIKE CRAZY. I WOULD ACTUALLY EAT THEM AS MOST WOULD EAT AN APPLE. AT THE TIME THEY SOME-HOW SEEMED KIND OF SWEET WITH A BIT OF A BITE AT THE SAME TIME. ALMOST LIKE JICAMA WITH A LITTLE CAYENNE TO IT. I HAD TO HAVE THEM WHENEVER THE CRAVING CAME. PROBABLY ATE ABOUT A TRUCK LOAD NO WAY I COULD DO IT NOW!

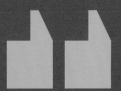

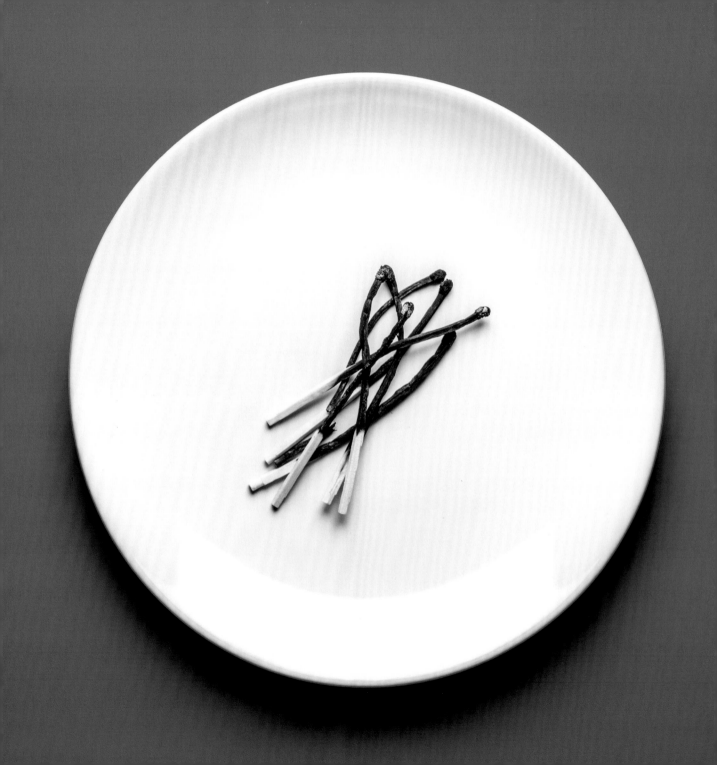

BURNT MATCHES

Kerry, Cape Town, South Africa

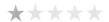

*The head tastes like garlicky egg and the rest tastes like nothing.
All in all, the experience isn't terrible. Unfortunately, the same can't be
said for your breath afterward.*

INGREDIENTS

One box of matches

METHOD

"Cook" the matches by burning them (preferably without setting off your smoke alarm).

SERVES 0—WE FELT OBLIGATED TO TRY THIS FOR ART, SCIENCE, AND YOUR AMUSEMENT. WE STRONGLY URGE YOU NOT TO BE SO MASOCHISTIC.

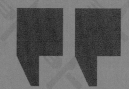

BURNT MATCHES

KERRY, CAPE TOWN, SOUTH AFRICA

The craving came out of nowhere when I was lighting a candle with a match. I always quite liked the smell of matches, but suddenly it smelled delicious and I was dying to taste it. It was the weirdest feeling. I remember holding the burnt match up to my nose and inhaling deeply. My mouth was watering, but there were other people around and I didn't want them to think I was nuts.

I couldn't stop thinking about it though, so when I was alone I lit another one and touched it with the tip of my tongue just to see what it was like. Before I knew it I was chewing on it. **IT WAS INDESCRIBABLY GOOD. I CARRIED A PERSONAL STASH OF MATCHES IN MY HANDBAG FROM THEN ON.** Although I ate them a lot, I always spat them out into a tissue instead of swallowing—I may be crazy but I'm not *that* crazy.

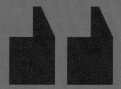

PEGGNUT BUTTER CUPS

Tina, West Liberty, Ohio, USA

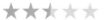

This unholy love child of a chicken and a peanut has the flavor of peanut butter, the texture of slimy rubber, and the appeal of a dad joke.

INGREDIENTS

2 eggs

2 tablespoons peanut butter

A few crushed peanuts

METHOD

Prick the eggs at the bottom and place inside a pot. Cover with water and bring to a boil over medium heat.

Let the eggs boil for 10–12 minutes.

Place the eggs in ice water to cool.

Peel the eggs and then cut in half lengthwise.

Remove the yolks with a teaspoon.

Put the peanut butter in a piping bag and pipe into the space where the yolk used to be.

Sprinkle the crushed peanut pieces onto the peanut butter.

Arrange on a plate and serve.

SERVES 1

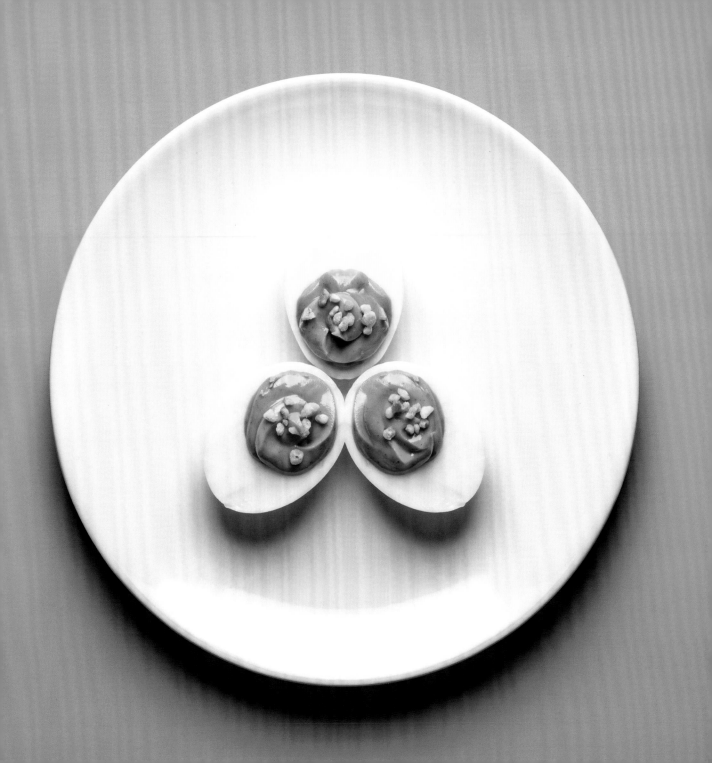

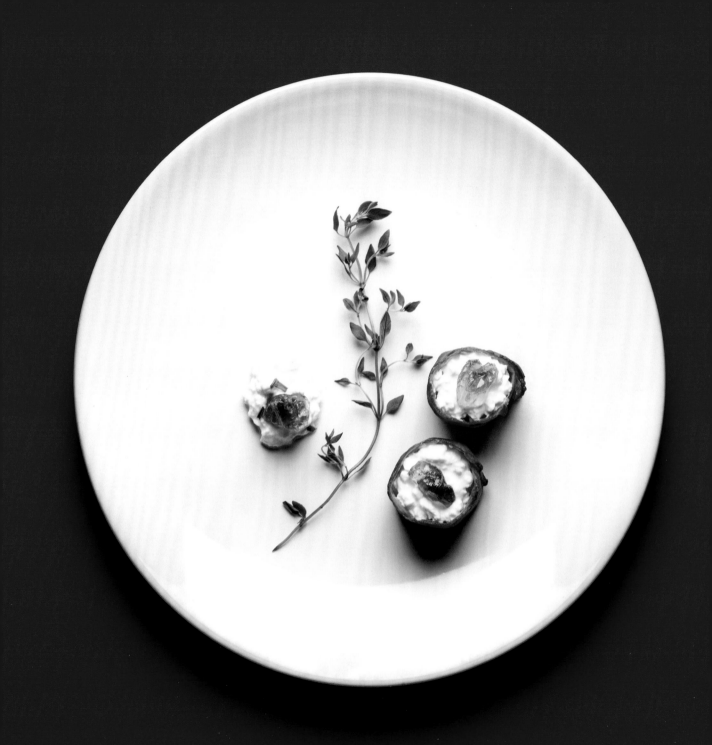

SWEET BACON AND COTTAGE CHEESE SUSHI ROLLS

Hannah, Hamburg, Germany

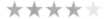

Proof that it doesn't matter what you wrap in bacon—cottage cheese, a worm, your shoe—it will still taste good.

INGREDIENTS

3 rashers of bacon

3 tablespoons cottage cheese

1 teaspoon brown sugar or 3 brown sugar crystals

METHOD

Preheat the oven to 250°F / 175°C.

Carefully roll each rasher of bacon around a 1-inch / 2-cm ring mold. Alternatively, you can squash a piece of tinfoil into a cylindrical shape and use that as your mold.

Grill in the oven for 10–15 minutes or until crispy.

Take out of the oven and let cool until you can safely handle the bacon and mold.

Slide the bacon off the mold and fill the center with cottage cheese.

Sprinkle the brown sugar on top of each roll.

SERVES 1

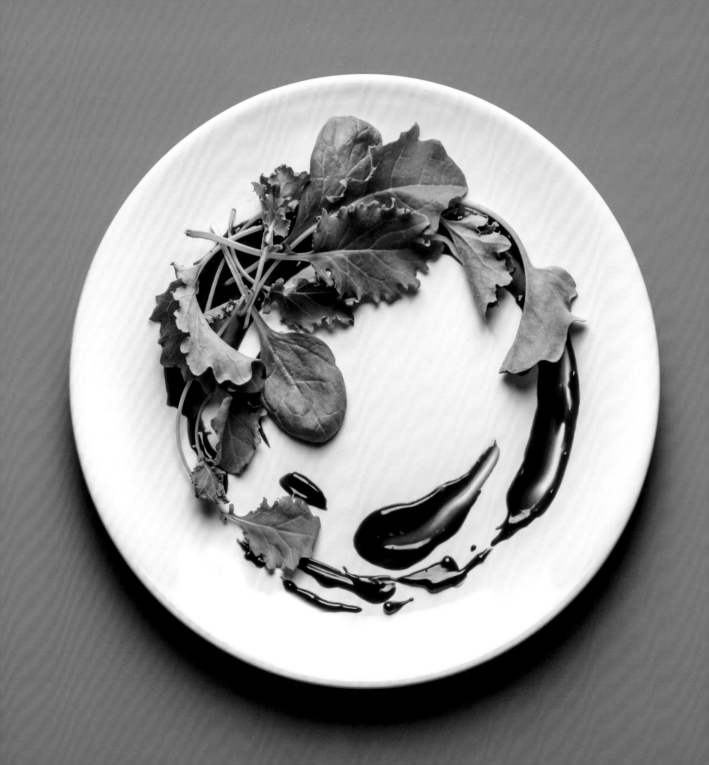

FORAGED GREENS WITH HOT FUDGE DRESSING

Maria João, Lisbon, Portugal

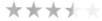

*Best results with a small portion of especially bland lettuce
and an extra serving of hot fudge.*

INGREDIENTS

¼ (14-ounce / 400-ml) can condensed milk

2 teaspoons cocoa powder (unsweetened)

1 tablespoon butter

⅛ teaspoon vanilla extract

2 ounces / 60 g salad mix

METHOD

Add the milk to a heavy saucepan and sift in the cocoa powder. Bring to a boil over medium heat, stirring frequently. Boil for 3 minutes while stirring constantly.

Remove the saucepan from the heat and add the butter. It should melt rapidly and can be stirred into the mixture.

Add the vanilla extract and stir.

While you wait for the hot fudge sauce to cool, wash the salad mix and pat dry with a paper towel.

Arrange the salad mix on a plate.

When the hot fudge is cool enough to eat, pour it artfully over the greens.

SERVES 1

STONE WALLS

Clair, Bristol, England

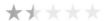

Tastes like expensive dental work.

INGREDIENTS

Cement wall

METHOD

Procure your piece of wall in the most legal way possible. Lick it or break off small, bite-size pieces.

SERVES 0—WE'LL MAKE YOU A DEAL. YOU DON'T EAT THIS. WE WON'T TELL YOUR NEIGHBORS WHAT YOU JUST DID TO THEIR WALL.

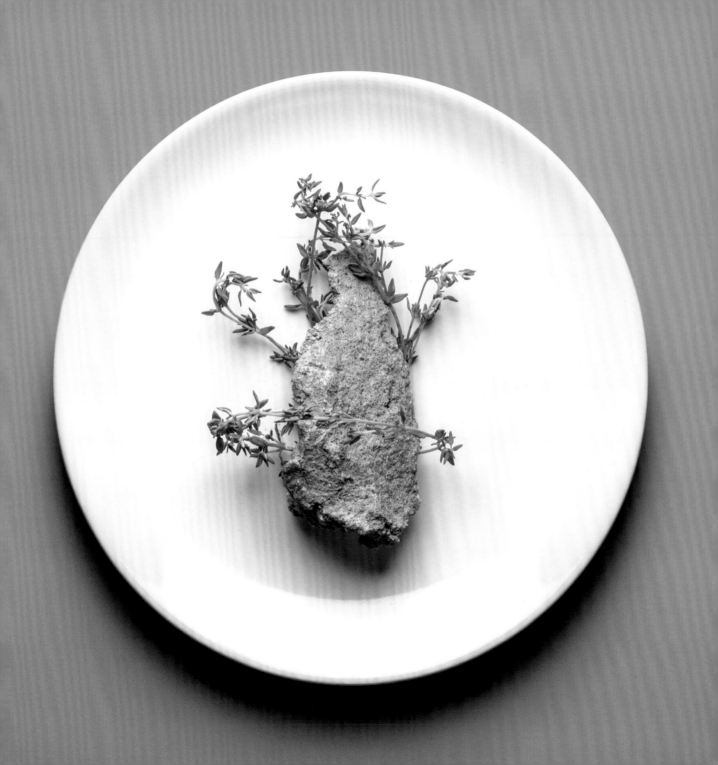

STONE
WALLS

CLAIR, BRISTOL, ENGLAND

I lived in a predominantly Victorian housing area. AS I WALKED PAST OLD BUILDINGS, THE SMELL OF DELICIOUS EARTHINESS WOULD BE IRRESISTIBLE. I would pick at the stone and collect little pieces to lick and crunch between my teeth. There was an old school wall that had a particularly crumbly texture that I liked to go to. Interestingly my mum had a craving for mud, the dried stuff that used to be left on potatoes when you brought them from the green grocers. She would lick the mud off the potatoes. So odd cravings seem to run in the family.

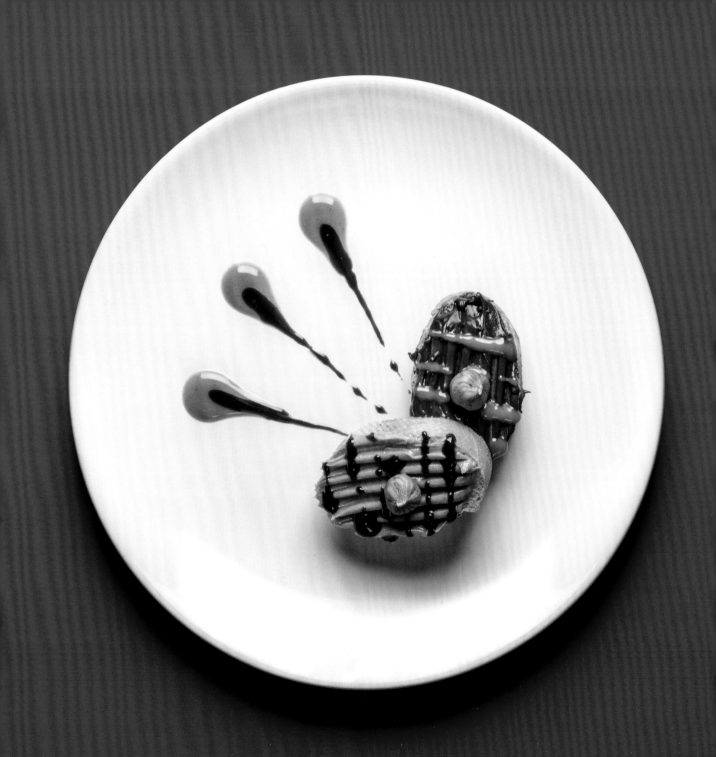

PEANUT BUTTER, BALSAMIC GLAZE, AND HAZELNUT SPREAD BITES

Margarita, Santander, Spain

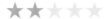

Everybody was having such a great time until the balsamic glaze came to the party.

INGREDIENTS

2 teaspoons hazelnut spread

2 slices of baguette

2 teaspoons peanut butter

1 teaspoon balsamic glaze

2 hazelnuts, for garnish

METHOD

Put a layer of hazelnut spread on one baguette slice, followed with a layer of peanut butter.

Use a fork to create an attractive pattern of lines.

Add a layer of balsamic glaze in stripes going in the opposite direction to the pattern created by the fork.

Repeat the process on the second slice of baguette, but change the order of the ingredients to create a color contrast. Top each bite with a hazelnut.

SERVES 1

POPCORN ON A BED OF SAUERKRAUT

Claudia, Hamburg, Germany

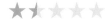

It's not any worse than sauerkraut by itself.

INGREDIENTS

1 (14-ounce / 400-ml) can of sauerkraut

1 bag of microwave popcorn

Sprig of thyme, for garnish

METHOD

Heat up the sauerkraut in a saucepan adding butter, salt, and pepper to taste.

Once it is warmed through, remove the saucepan from the heat.

Follow the instructions on the packet of the microwave popcorn. Be careful to note which side is "up."

Place a portion of the sauerkraut on a plate. Add some of the popcorn on top, garnish with thyme, and serve.

SERVES 1 VERY HUNGRY PERSON.

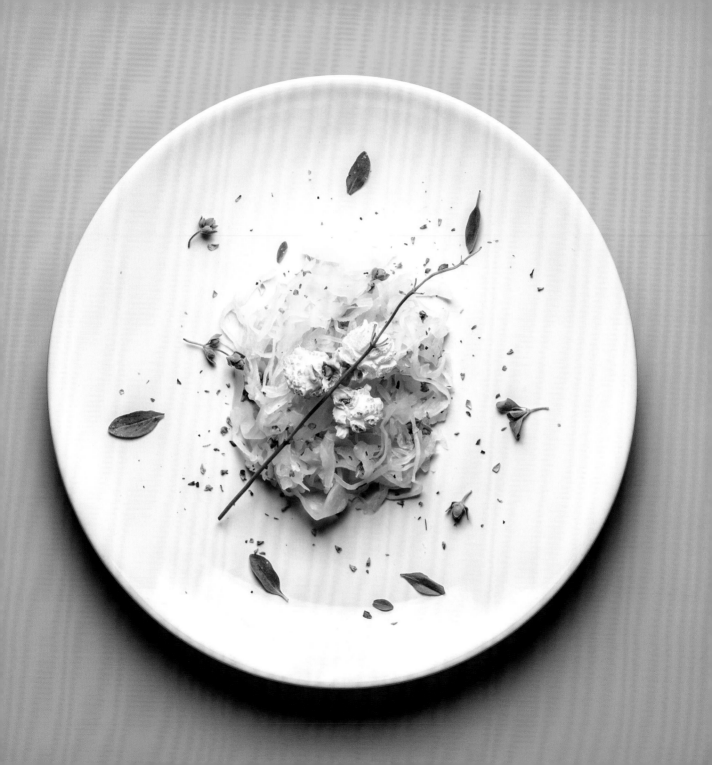

RAW BROCCOLI WITH APPLESAUCE

Sara, Gahanna, Ohio, USA

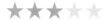

*A little weird but inoffensive and instantly forgettable.
If "meh" was a flavor it would probably be broccoli with applesauce.*

INGREDIENTS

1 apple

1 tablespoon brown sugar

3 tablespoons water

1 stick cinnamon

1 cup small broccoli florets,
uncooked

METHOD

Peel the apple, core it, and cut into pieces, leaving two slices to use later as garnish.

Add the apples to a saucepan with the sugar, water, and cinnamon and allow the mixture to simmer over medium heat for about 15 minutes.

When the apples are soft, remove the saucepan from the heat and allow to cool.

Remove the cinnamon stick, retaining it to use as a garnish, then puree the mixture until smooth.

Serve the raw broccoli with the applesauce.

Garnish with the remaining apple slices and the cinnamon stick.

SERVES 1

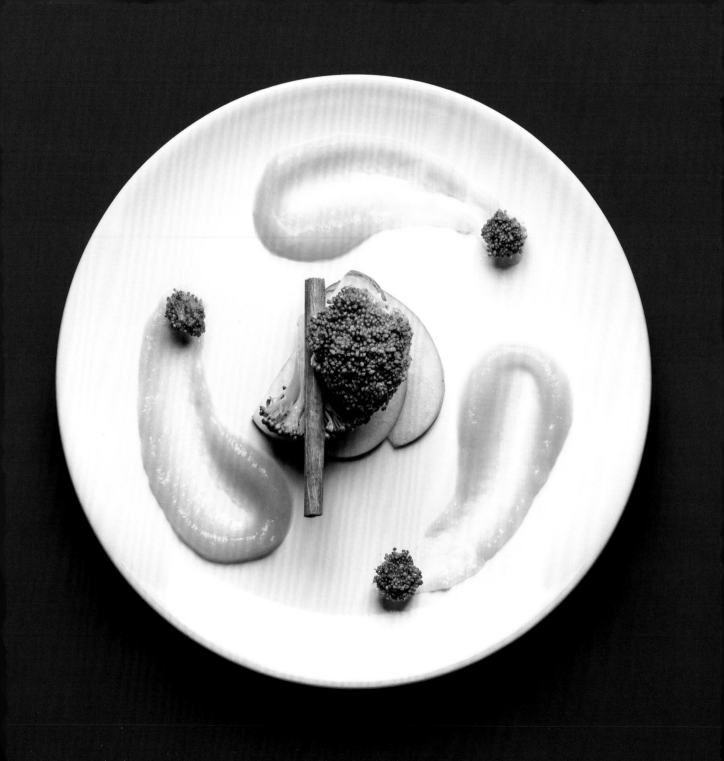

RAW BROCCOLI WITH APPLESAUCE

SARA, GAHANNA, OHIO, USA

The craving sort of hit me out of nowhere. I was about fourteen weeks along and I had just gotten out of the shower. As I walked down the stairs I felt like I got a whiff of apples and for whatever reason, I immediately decided that broccoli was the absolute best thing to add to applesauce. I wanted something crunchy and smooth so **I DECIDED TO JUST BREAK THE RAW BROCCOLI INTO FLORETS AND DIP THEM IN THE APPLESAUCE. LIKE CHIPS AND SALSA, ONLY HEALTHIER AND TASTING NOTHING LIKE CHIPS OR SALSA.**

My son, who was seven years old then, tried it once but hated it. He got in the habit of sitting by me with a spoon when I ate it so he could steal the applesauce. When I told my mom about it, the next time I visited her, she had broccoli and applesauce there for me. It was so sweet.

I remember eating it once every two or three days until the sixth month when I developed an intense craving for burnt popcorn . . . something I still eat today, three years later.

But I did try it again when my daughter was probably eight months old and was showing a sudden aversion to breast milk so I started eating my favorite pregnant foods to help familiarize the flavor for her. I wasn't as enthusiastic about the combination after birth, but my daughter had no problem nursing after that!

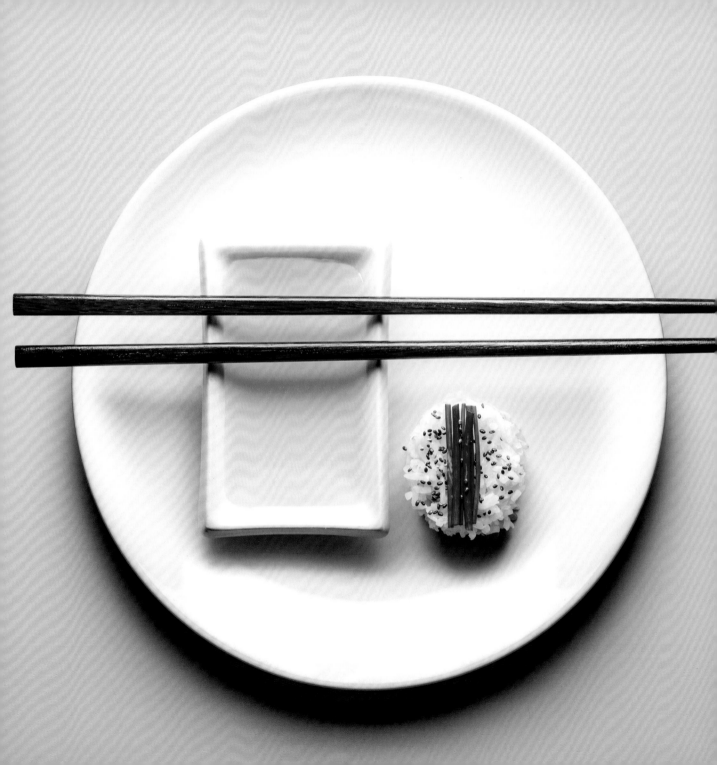

RICE AND GASOLINE

Maria, Vespasiano, Minas Gerais, Brazil

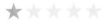

*Reviewed like a fine wine because it was sampled like a fine wine:
sniffed, tasted, then spat out. The bouquet was a bitch-slap of toxic fumes.
Distinctive notes of spicy ink dominated the flavor, leading to a
hard-to-rinse-out finish tinged with regret.*

INGREDIENTS

¼ cup / 65 g rice

¼ cup / 60 ml gasoline

METHOD

Rinse the rice until the water runs clear.

Add ½ cup / 120 ml water and a pinch of salt.

Stir once, then bring to a boil.

Simmer on low heat for about 15 minutes or until cooked.

Remove the rice from the heat and drain well.

Serve the rice onto a plate and either pour the gasoline over it or put it next to the rice in a dipping bowl.

SERVES 0—NO! ARE YOU NUTS?
PUT THE CHOPSTICKS DOWN.

BBQ BEETS

Jessica, Adelaide, Australia

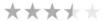

A juicy, tasty mess. It's the innovative new salad for people to ignore at your next BBQ.

INGREDIENTS

1 beet

1–2 tablespoons BBQ sauce

METHOD

Wash the beet, being careful not to tear the skin, and then trim the top and root. Be sure not to cut too much off or the color will bleed into the water.

Put in a pot of water and bring to a boil.

Simmer on low heat for about 25 minutes.

Drain into a colander and allow to cool slightly.

Slice the beet into even slices, arrange into a fan, and pour the BBQ sauce on top.

SERVES 1

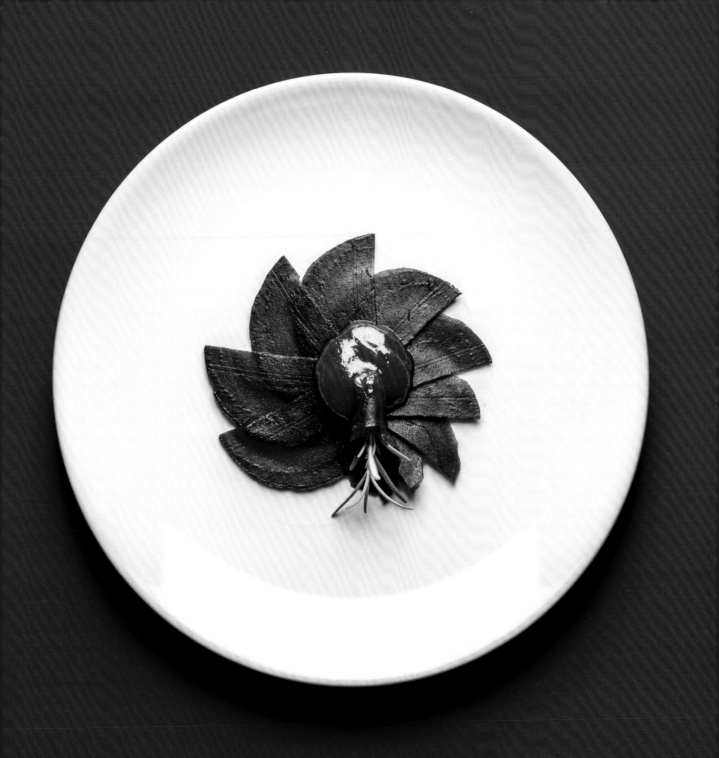

BBQ BEETS

JESSICA, ADELAIDE, AUSTRALIA

When I was pregnant, I truly thought this was the greatest thing I had ever eaten. BEING PREVIOUSLY TRAINED AS A CHEF I HAD TASTED MY FAIR SHARE OF CULINARY DELIGHTS BUT THIS ONE TOPPED THEM ALL!

My strange craving came about when I was hungry. I knew I hadn't been eating the best so I was thinking about something healthy. A salad sandwich came to mind. I wasn't so sure about the lettuce, though. Maybe just bread, cheese, BBQ sauce, cucumber, and BEET-ROOT! I already love beetroot but as soon as the word had entered my head I had to have it NOW! Forget the rest of the sandwich. That amazing earthy flavor. I still wanted the BBQ sauce though and thus my strange craving was born. I ate it every day for lunch for weeks, sometimes more than once and snacked on it throughout the day. I had to have at least one tin of beetroot a day minimum.

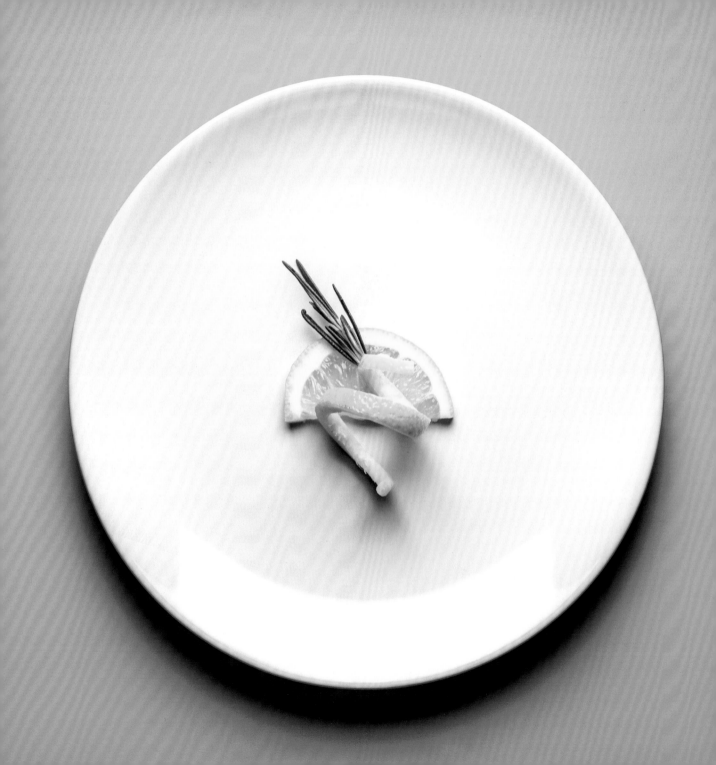

LEMONS WITH SKIN

Kate, Cedar Lake, Indiana, USA

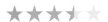

*The dish has a lemony aroma and a lemony taste intensified by
the lemony lemon peel and lemony aftertaste.*

INGREDIENTS

METHOD

1 lemon

Wash the lemon well.

Cut it in half lengthwise and then into slices about
½ inch / 1 cm thick.

When eating, do not discard the skin, but eat it with the rest
of the fruit.

SERVES 1

LEMONS WITH SKIN

KATE, CEDAR LAKE, INDIANA, USA

I GOT THE IDEA FOR THE "RECIPE" ONLY BECAUSE I WAS CRAVING LEMONS SO BADLY AND WAS FINDING WAYS TO INCORPORATE THEM ANYWAY I COULD. I LOVED THE SMELL AND THE TEXTURE. MY FAMILY THOUGHT I WAS CRAZY WALKING AROUND WITH LEMONS ALL THE TIME BUT DID NOT COMPLAIN AT HOW FRESH I ALWAYS SMELLED.

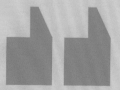

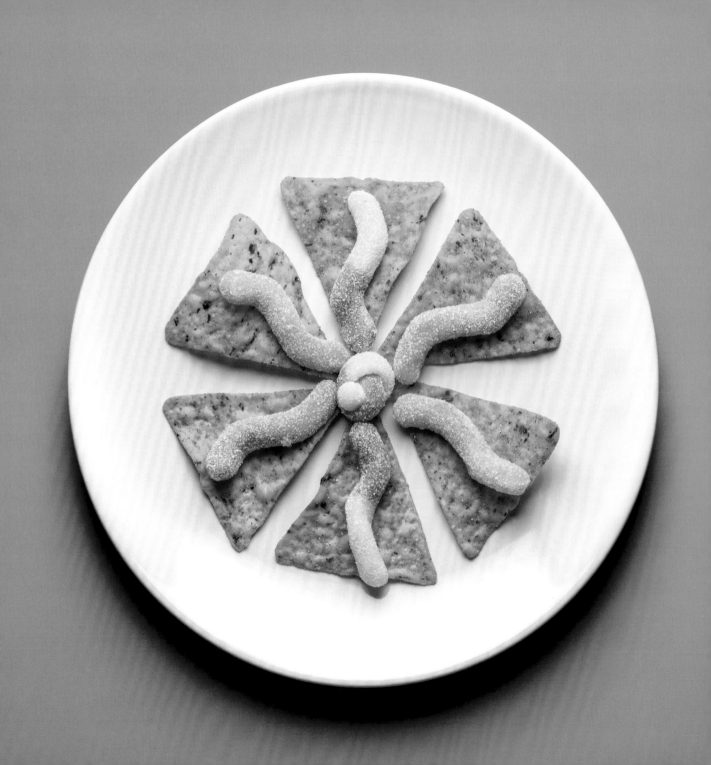

CHIPS AND SOUR GUMMI WORMS

Meryl, Johannesburg, South Africa

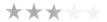

It's not so much bad as unnecessary. Like a Romeo and Juliet sequel.

INGREDIENTS

6 nacho cheese tortilla chips

*6 sour gummi worms
(about 1 small bag)*

METHOD

Arrange the chips on a plate and put a sour gummi worm on top of each chip.

———————

SERVES 1

TOMATO SOUP WITH M&MS

Nicole, Thomasville, North Carolina, USA

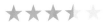

*The kind of thing you might end up eating if you forgot to go shopping
and have no food at home. That, or you are really stoned.*

INGREDIENTS

¼ white onion, finely chopped

1 tablespoon olive oil

1½ cups / 240 g chopped
fresh tomatoes

⅔ cup / 160 ml chicken stock

1 teaspoon sugar

Pinch of salt

1 tablespoon chopped
fresh parsley

¼ cup / 60 ml heavy cream

Optional: 1 teaspoon sherry

Pepper

5–10 different-colored M&Ms

METHOD

Fry the onions in the olive oil until translucent.

Add the tomatoes, stock, sugar, salt, and parsley.

Simmer on medium heat for 20 minutes.

Allow to cool a little and then puree the mixture until smooth.

Return to the pot and add the cream, sherry (if desired),
and pepper to taste.

Serve in a bowl and sprinkle the M&Ms on top like croutons.

SERVES 1

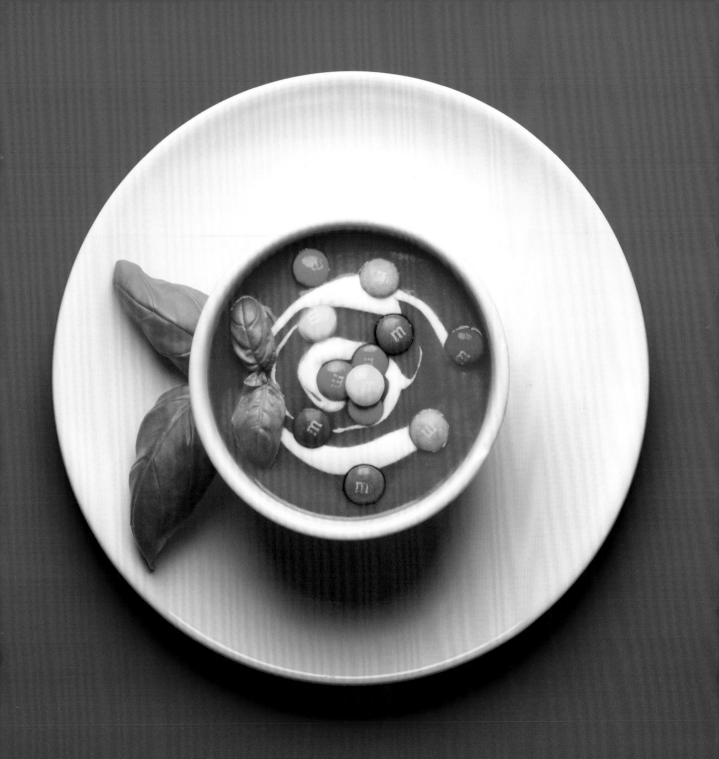

TOMATO SOUP WITH M&MS

NICOLE, THOMASVILLE, NORTH CAROLINA, USA

The idea honestly just popped into my head as I was sitting at work answering phones. My job was at a resort, and the kitchen staff was extremely helpful during my pregnancy. They made a lunch "special" for me. When I first tried it, this weird feeling of full body satisfaction occurred. The taste was wonderful while pregnant . . . a good combination of bitter and sweet. It was my midnight snack for at least a month.

My entire family thought I was crazy and would usually make puking noises with every spoonful. MY NOW SCHOOL-AGED SON GIGGLES EVERY TIME I TELL HIM ABOUT THAT CRAVING. When asked if he would ever try it, he just says, "Ew, Momma. Never!"

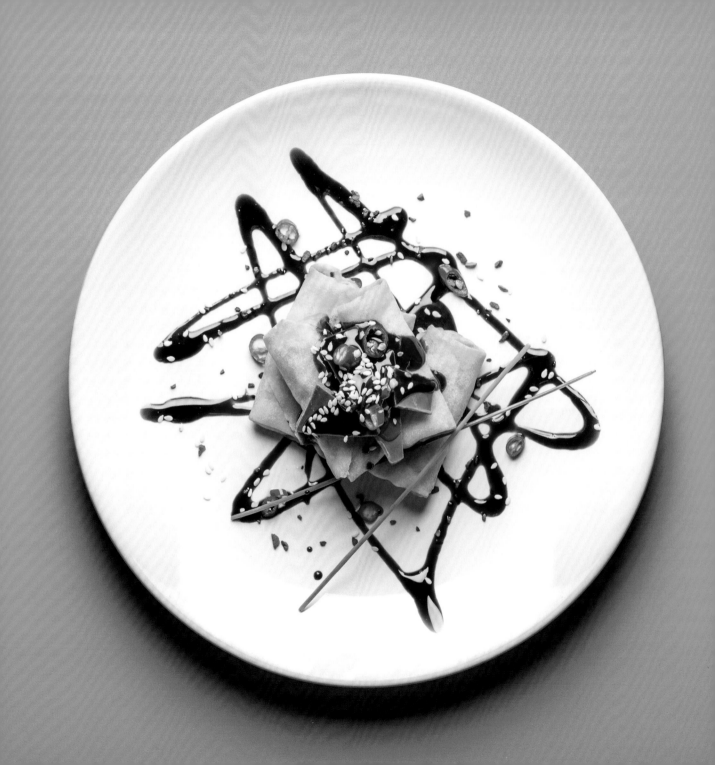

SPRING ROLLS WITH CHOCOLATE SAUCE

Jenny, Johannesburg, South Africa

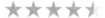

You have been eating spring rolls wrong all your life.
If Einstein was a cook, this is the recipe he would have come up with.

INGREDIENTS

6 frozen mini spring rolls

3 ounces / 90 ml store-bought chocolate sauce

½ small red chile pepper, chopped, for garnish

METHOD

Heat the spring rolls according to package directions.

Arrange in a stack on a plate.

Dribble chocolate sauce over the spring rolls generously.

Serve.

Add the chile pepper for garnish.

_____

SERVES 1

TOILET PAPER

Kelli, Los Angeles, USA

....

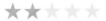

There are no surprises here. It is exactly what you would expect eating toilet paper is like. And also exactly why it is made for your butt and not your mouth.

....

INGREDIENTS

1 roll of toilet paper
Water

METHOD

There are many different methods for preparing toilet paper. This is the "Classic Rose" method.

Set up a small bowl of water to dip your fingers in to style the toilet paper.

Unroll the paper until you have approximately sixteen squares in a strip.

Tear off the strip and scrunch it together until it forms something similar to a rose.

Sprinkle a little water on one side to hold the shape and place it on a plate.

Tear eight individual squares of toilet paper off the roll.

Dampen each one and roll into a ball.

Arrange the balls of toilet paper around your rose.

_____

SERVES 0—OH, YOU ACTUALLY TOOK THE TIME TO MAKE THIS? SORRY, NO, YOU CAN'T EAT IT. AND YOU CAN'T GET THOSE 15 MINUTES OF YOUR LIFE BACK, EITHER.

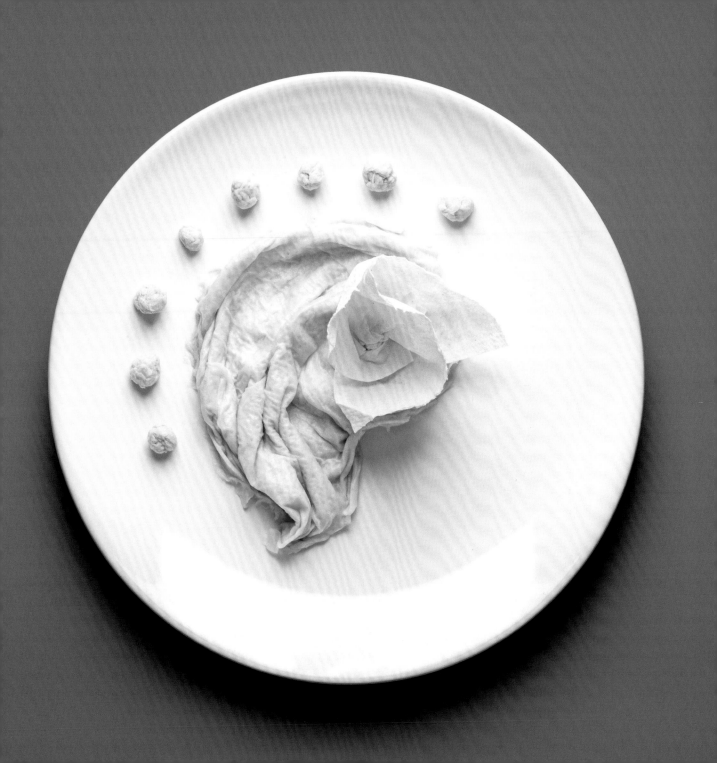

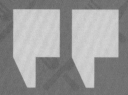

TOILET
PAPER

KELLI, LOS ANGELES, USA

It started with me noticing the smell of it. Sometimes it smelled sweet and then other days it smelled like a real musty old bus. And the weird thing was I wanted to eat it more when it smelled like a bus!

I only tried it a few times as I was scared I was clogging myself up but I liked the texture and flavor. IT KIND OF TASTED LIKE CANDY FLOSS AT FIRST AND THEN ONCE IT WAS ALL CHEWED AND MASHED IT LOST ITS FLAVOR AND JUST TASTED HORRIBLE. Like when you have a tooth out and the doctor shoves a cotton wool ball in your mouth.

It started with a square at a time until that wasn't doing anything for me. The most I ate at one time was about twenty squares. I know, pregnancy makes you do strange things.

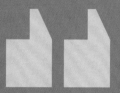

CRAB STICKS WITH JAM

Camilla, Xanxerê, Santa Catarina, Brazil

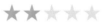

This wouldn't be half bad if you replaced the crabs with a hamburger patty and the jam with some ketchup . . . maybe added a bun, some cheese, bacon, and French fries and a Coke . . .

INGREDIENTS

2 crab sticks

1 chive to use as a tie

1 tablespoon alfalfa sprouts

1 tablespoon jam of your choice (we used rose petal)

METHOD

Remove the crab sticks from the packaging.

Tie them together using one long chive.

Place on a bed of sprouts.

Dribble jam on top and around artistically.

_____

SERVES 1

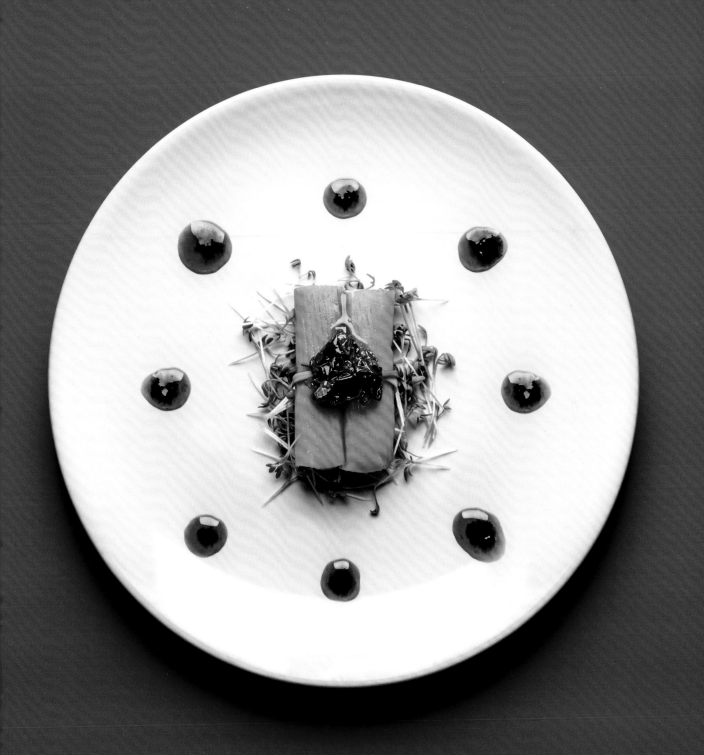

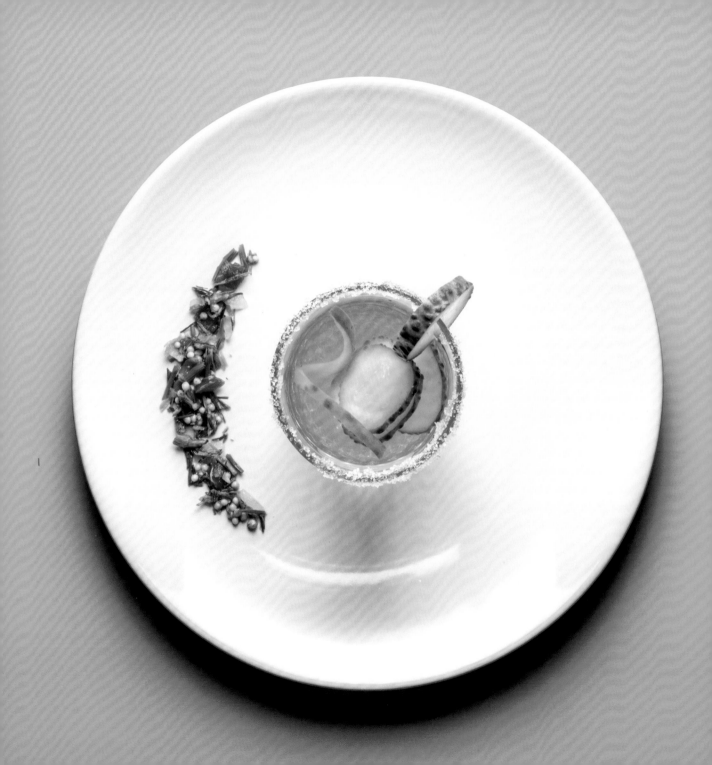

PICKLE COCKTAIL

Roseanne, West Islip, New York, USA

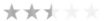

It tastes like a cup of diluted salad dressing. Not really so bad, but not the type of thing you would drink given a choice of . . . well . . . anything else ever.

INGREDIENTS

1 bottle of pickles

METHOD

Pour the juice from the bottle of pickles into a glass.

Add some slices or whole pickles for decoration.

Use the seasoning from the pickle bottle as garnish.

Drink.

SERVES 1

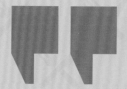

PICKLE
COCKTAIL

ROSEANNE, WEST ISLIP, NY, USA

IT WAS BASICALLY THE BEST DRINK I'VE EVER HAD. IT'S SO SATISFYING IN SUCH A STRANGE WAY. I WOULD DRINK IT AS OFTEN AS I HAD PICKLES IN THE HOUSE. MY HUSBAND AND MOTHER WOULD GET MAD BECAUSE THE PICKLES WOULD DRY OUT. BUT MY SON WOULD DANCE AROUND INSIDE ME WHEN I DRANK IT SO I GUESS HE LIKED IT, TOO!

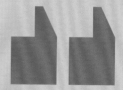

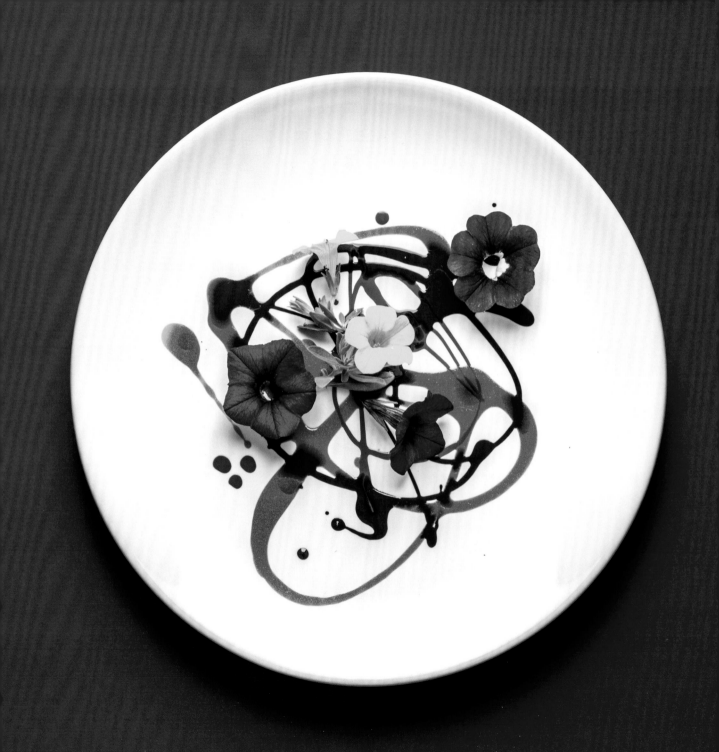

NAIL POLISH

Nino, Tbilisi, Georgia

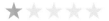

It tastes like spicy fire. With an aftertaste of swearing, spitting, and mouth-washing.

INGREDIENTS

1–5 different colored nail polishes

METHOD

Open the bottles and pour onto a plate in aesthetically pleasing shapes.

Decorate with some flowers that complement your nail polish colors.

SERVES 0—GO TO THE TRASH. GO DIRECTLY TO THE TRASH. DO NOT PASS BY THE MOUTH. DO NOT COLLECT $200 WORTH OF MEDICAL BILLS.

NAIL
POLISH

NINO, TBILISI, GEORGIA

I WAS ADDICTED TO ALL STRONG CHEMICAL SMELLS LIKE GASOLINE AND HOUSEHOLD CLEANING PRODUCTS. BUT NAIL POLISH WAS MY FAVORITE. I ONLY ACTUALLY TASTED IT ONCE—IT WAS QUITE POTENT BUT IN A GOOD WAY. AND I HAVE TO SAY, MY NAILS NEVER LOOKED BETTER THAN WHEN I WAS PREGNANT!

"

HOT DOGS WITH PEANUT BUTTER DIP

Nikki, San Diego, California, USA

★★☆☆☆

The first time being allergic to nuts will work out to your advantage.

INGREDIENTS

2 tablespoons peanut butter

1–3 hot dogs

METHOD

Place peanut butter in a small dish.

Dip hot dogs into the peanut butter and eat.

_____

SERVES 1

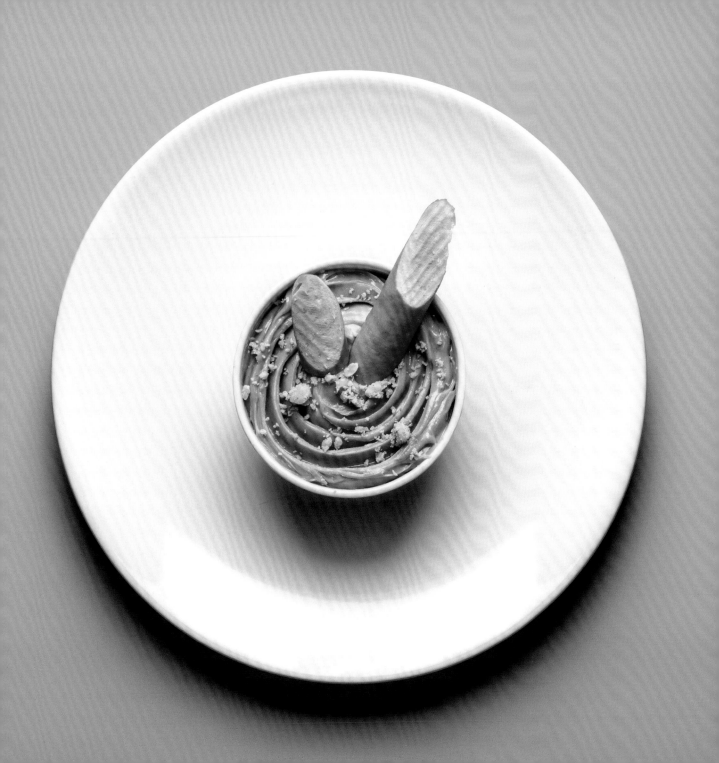

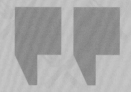

HOT DOGS WITH PEANUT BUTTER DIP

NIKKI, SAN DIEGO, CALIFORNIA, USA

Basically I craved peanut butter but didn't want the sweet taste people pair it with, like fresh fruit or jelly. I wanted something salty and hot. I would try to play it off and eat a bite of apple dipped in peanut butter followed by a bite of hot dog. One day, I ran out of apple. So I did what I finally wanted to and I dipped my hot dog in the peanut butter and took a giant bite. It was delicious!

I HAVE LEARNED THAT WEIRD FLAVORS PASS ON! MY OLDEST TWO CHILDREN ARE OBSESSED WITH PEANUT BUTTER, and adore putting cheese on their PB&Js! I'm actually pregnant with my third and can't stand peanut butter now, though.

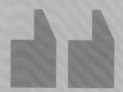

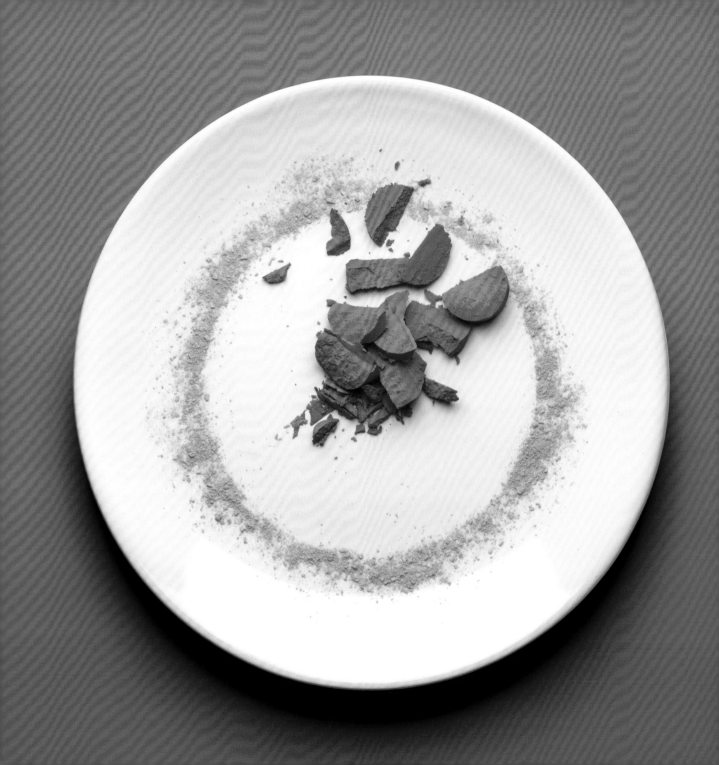

CHALK

Elmira, Cork, Ireland

....

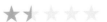

*That horrifying moment when you realize that "melt in your mouth"
texture has an evil twin. A really, really evil twin.*

....

INGREDIENTS

*2 large pieces of chalk in different
colors, e.g., green and red*

METHOD

Grate the green chalk into powder.

Put a smaller bowl on your plate and sprinkle green powder
around it to create a circle.

Put the red chalk in the middle of the plate and slice
into pieces.

———————————

SERVES 0—IF YOU ARE CRAVING THIS, PLEASE
CALL YOUR DOCTOR. IF YOU AREN'T BUT WANT TO
TRY IT ANYWAY, PLEASE CALL YOUR THERAPIST.
EITHER WAY, DON'T TRY THIS AT HOME.

SANDY CHIPS

Treys, Windsor, Ontario, Canada

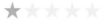

*Those grains of sand are like vicious little ninjas. They wreak havoc
in your mouth, then go into hiding, only to reappear when you least expect it with
a hideous, tooth-breaking crunch.*

INGREDIENTS

2 ounces / 56 g sand

1 ounce / 28 g potato chips

METHOD

There are various methods to create this dish, the simplest of which is just to pour some sand into a bag of chips and shake.

Pictured is the sand-stripe version. Carefully pour lines of sand onto your plate.

Place chips across the lines at regular intervals.

Finish off by sprinkling a little sand on top of the chips.

SERVES 0—SINCE YOU REALLY SHOULDN'T EAT THIS, IT'S A BIT OF A SAD WASTE OF CHIPS.

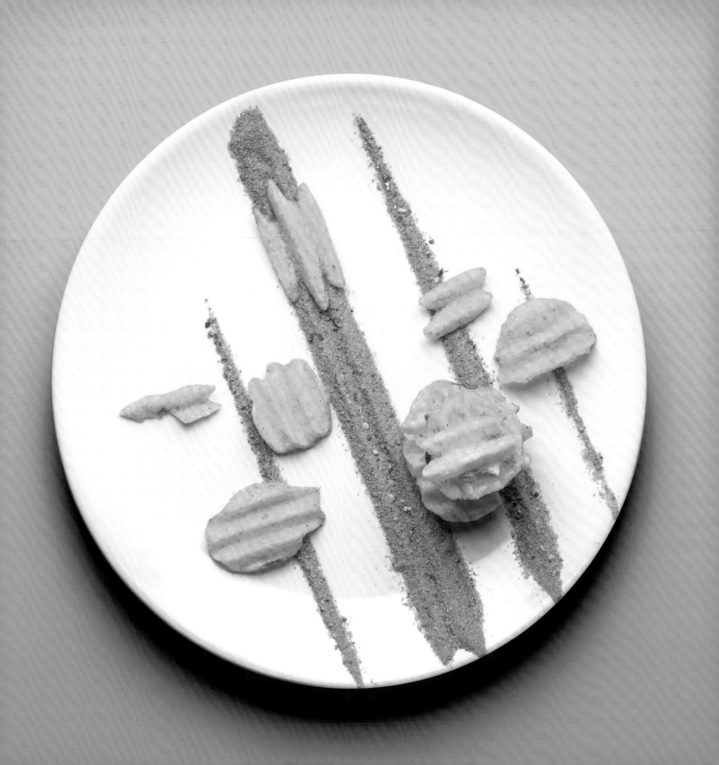

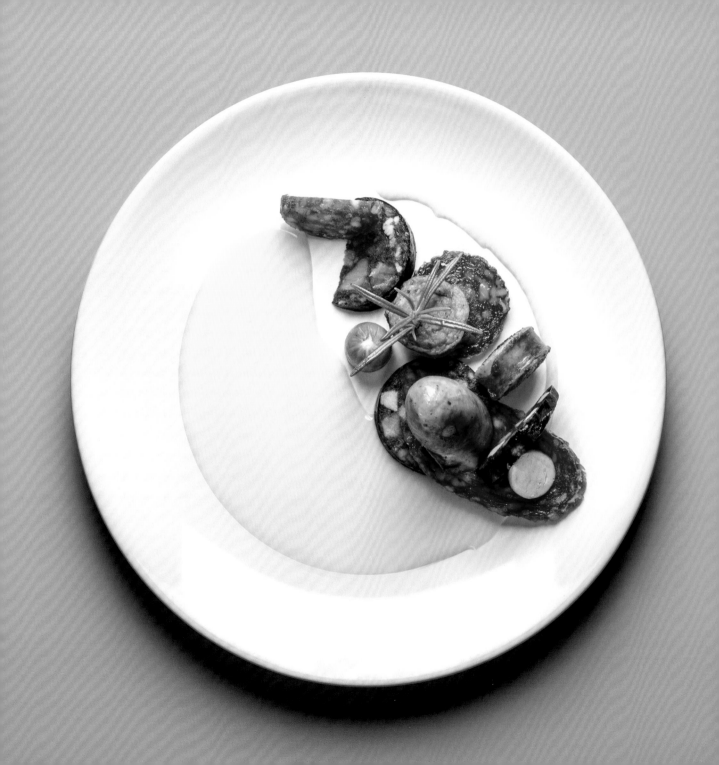

SALAMI AND CONDENSED MILK

Francisca, Panamá, Goiás, Brazil

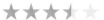

*This dish is actually surprisingly tasty, but there just seems
no place for it in the world. Too common for a restaurant.
Too unhealthy to give the kids. Too weird to eat alone. Too much shame at
the bottom of a can of condensed milk.*

INGREDIENTS

*1 salami (or ¼ each of four
different types of salami if you are
looking for a bit of variety)*

*¼ (14-ounce / 400-ml) can
condensed milk*

METHOD

Slice the salami into thin slices.

Place on a plate and pour the milk around it.

Eat by dipping each piece of salami into the milk.

———————————

SERVES 1

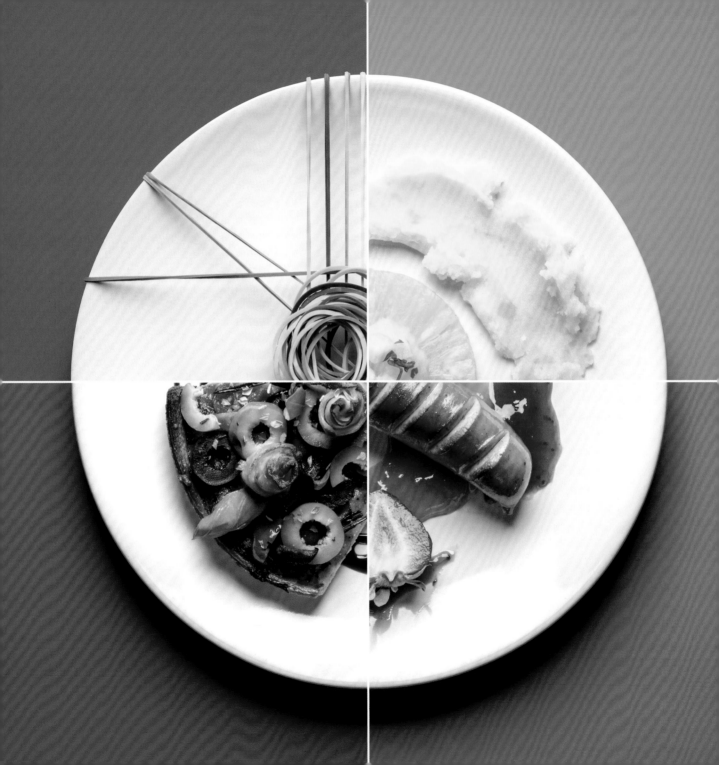

MAINS

While you can make a main course out of any craving if you eat enough of it, this chapter is a collection of the heartier dishes more likely to fill you up. Some very creative variations on burgers, meats, and sides await. As well as one or two very creative variations on the concept of food.

The very first recipe in this chapter, we are proud to say, was taste-tested by not only us but the (now adult) son of the woman who craved it when pregnant with him. His reaction? "Now I know why I turned out so weird."

LEMON AND CHOCOLATE PRAWNS ON A BED OF SPINACH

Maria, Lisbon, Portugal

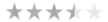

Quite tasty. Especially after you have tried some of the other recipes and your standards have been lowered.

INGREDIENTS

1 tablespoon butter

½ clove garlic, crushed

1–5 raw king prawns with shells

2½ ounces / 70 g fresh spinach

2 tablespoons olive oil

Pinch of salt

Pinch of pepper

¼ lemon

1 ounce / 30 g chocolate

1 slice of lemon

METHOD

On medium heat, melt the butter and fry the crushed garlic for about a minute.

Add the prawns and cook, turning occasionally until they have turned pink (approximately 5–8 minutes). If you are pregnant make extra-sure they are well cooked.

Remove from the pan and reserve.

Wash and de-stem the spinach.

Heat the olive oil in the same pan that was used to fry the prawns.

Add the washed, de-stemmed spinach and stir fry for about 2 minutes. Add salt and pepper.

Arrange a bed of spinach on the plate and put the prawns on top.

Squeeze the lemon over the dish.

Crush the chocolate into smaller pieces then add the chocolate and lemon slice.

Serve.

SERVES 1

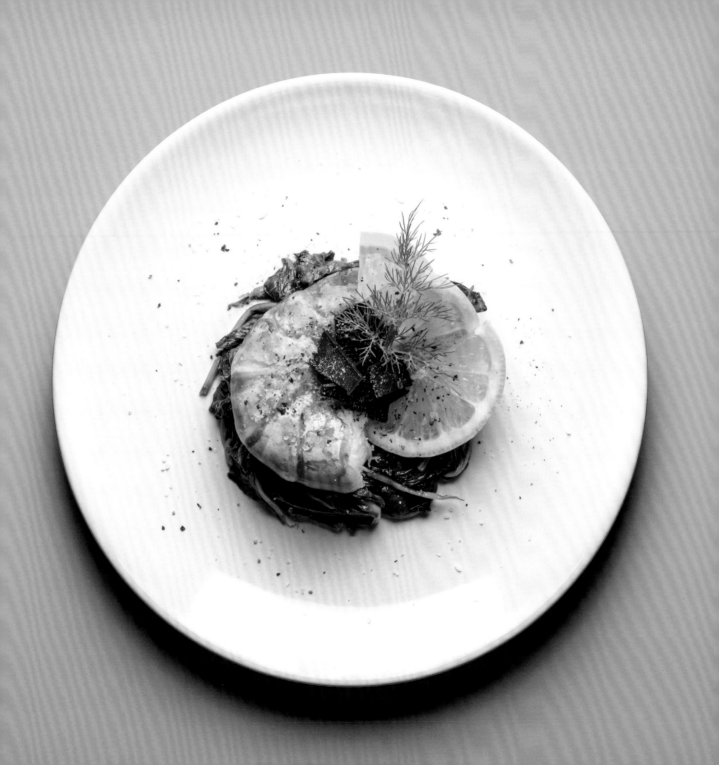

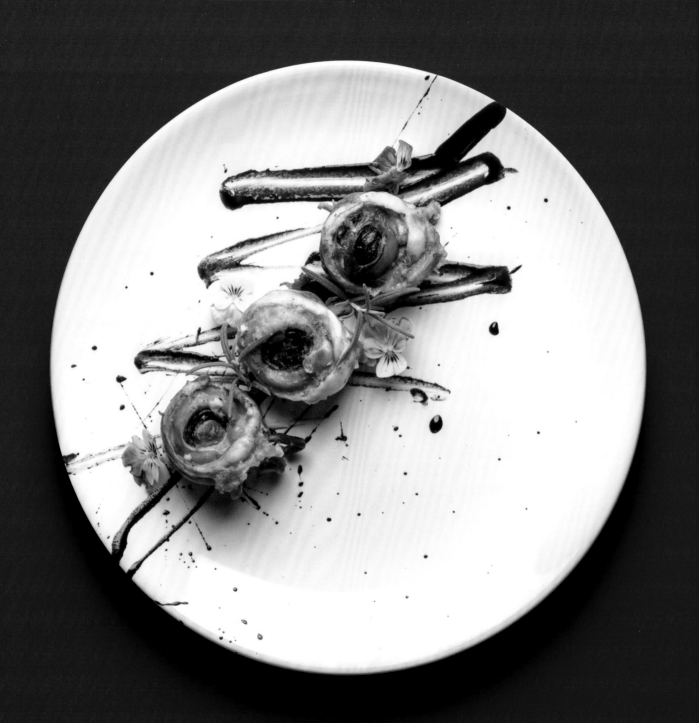

LAMB'S EYES

Danielle, Johannesburg, South Africa

★★★★★

Let us never speak of this again.

INGREDIENTS

3 lamb's eyes

Olive oil

Salt

Pepper

Rosemary

METHOD

Preheat the oven to 200ºC / 400ºF.

Brush the eyes with some olive oil, sprinkle with salt, pepper, and rosemary, and roast for about 20 minutes.

When plating, feel free to add some red wine sauce, rosemary, and edible flowers as we did because why the hell not.

SERVES 1 VERY UNLUCKY PERSON

LAMB'S EYES

DANIELLE, JOHANNESBURG, SOUTH AFRICA

I became a vegetarian at the age of fifteen. The big pity for me was, however, that my taste buds and consuming passions were in direct conflict with my moral sensibilities—I had always loved, and I mean really, really loved, meat. In the end, I settled on being a pescatarian, and had been happily eating that way for about twenty years. All of this changed, however, when, at the age of thirty-six, I fell pregnant with my son. I had dreamt of a glorious, raw, vegetarian pregnancy, and imagined my body rejecting anything that was unclean. Instead, all that I wanted to eat was chocolate and—driven by an increasingly irrepressible animal craving—meat. I managed to hold myself back, virtuously sticking to salads and veggies, stuffing fresh fruit into my ravenous face, but found it increasingly difficult to ignore my body's all-too-clear message that what it wanted was animal fat and blood.

I was five months pregnant when we went on holiday to Morocco and my cravings hit fever pitch whilst walking through the famously fabulous Marrakesh market. My feral nose—filled with the scents of every possible creature's every possible body part being cooked in every possible way—led me to a display of roasted lamb's heads, whose shiny, gooey eyeballs glowed at me, offering me the promise of tastes and sensations that would transport me into a state of pregnant bliss. **AS I LUNGED TOWARDS THE LAMB'S HEAD, LITERALLY ABOUT TO STICK MY FINGERS INTO THE ORIFICES TO EXTRACT AND DEVOUR THE DRIPPING ORBS, MY PARTNER YANKED ME BACK IN HORROR, ASKING ME WHAT THE HELL I THOUGHT I WAS DOING,** just as my virtue-mechanisms snapped into place to stop me. I never tasted the eyeballs.

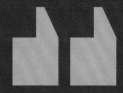

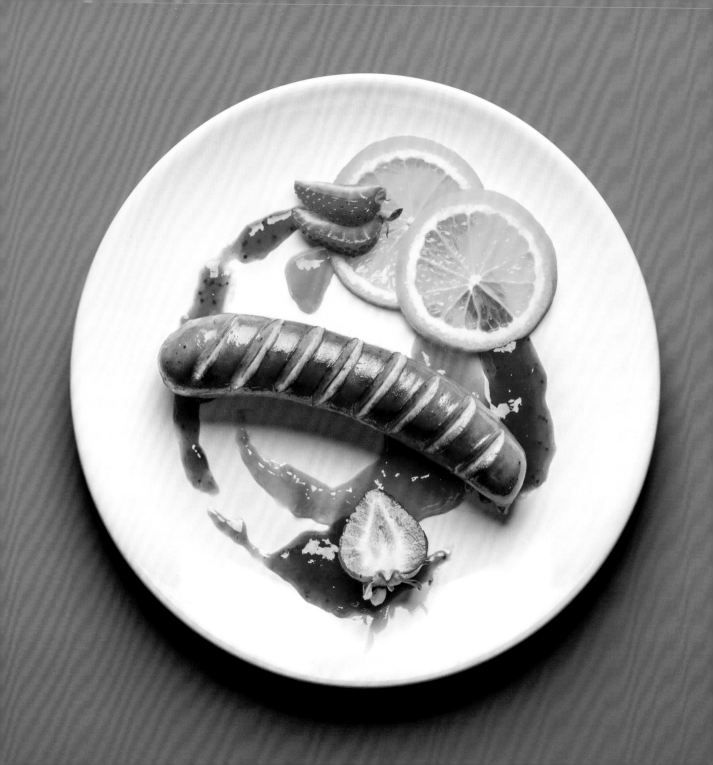

SAUSAGE AND JAM

Valerie, Folkestone, Kent, England

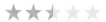

We had high hopes for this one. So you could say, this is what disappointment tastes like.

INGREDIENTS

1 sausage

1 tablespoon strawberry jam

1 tablespoon apricot marmalade

METHOD

Fry the sausage in a hot pan until it is brown and crispy on all sides.

Eat using the jam as a sauce.

———————

SERVES 1

BANANA-AND-PEANUT-BUTTER-STUFFED JALAPEÑOS

Brandi, Jamestown, North Dakota, USA

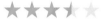

*Banana-peanut-butter-stuffed jalapeños has thirty-seven letters.
"This is the worst-tasting thing in this book" also has thirty-seven letters.
Coincidence? Yes, actually. The worst-tasting thing in this book is the Lamb's Eyes
on page 89. This is actually pretty darn good.*

INGREDIENTS

1 jalapeño pepper

2 teaspoons peanut butter

¼ banana

3 or 4 peanuts, crushed

METHOD

Slice the jalapeño pepper lengthwise in half.

Remove the white flesh and seeds so that there is a hollow cavity. Reserve seeds if you enjoy spicy food.

Stuff the pepper with the peanut butter.

Cut the banana into squares about ¼ inch / ½ cm in size and place them on top.

Crush the peanuts and sprinkle on top.

Add a few jalapeño seeds if you want to add a bit of extra bite.

———————

SERVES 1

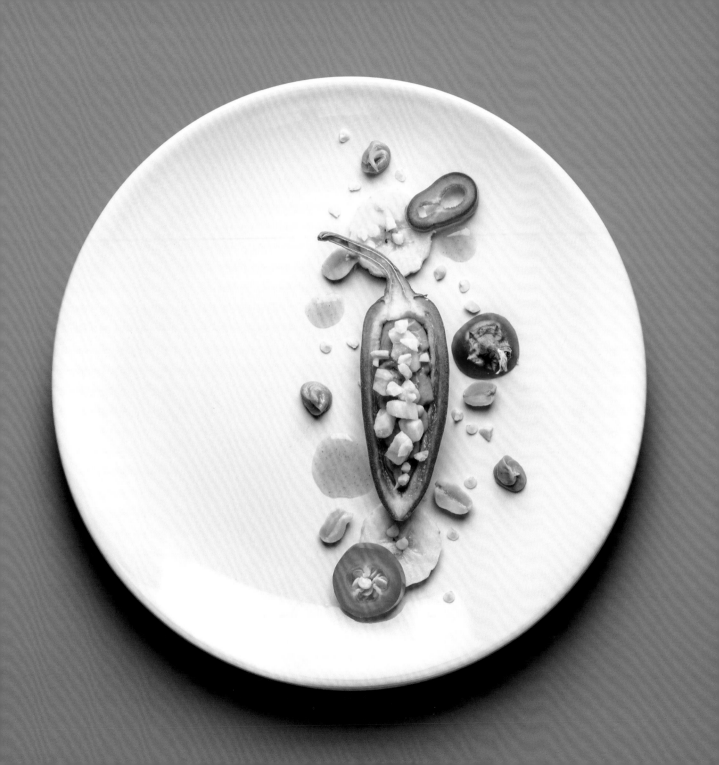

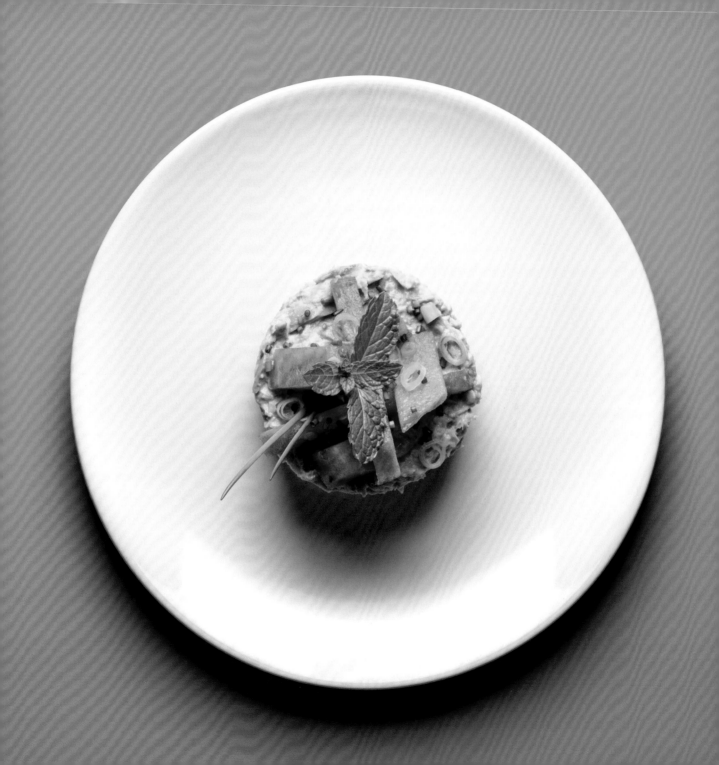

TUNA MAYO-MELON

Scarlett, Dallas–Fort Worth, USA

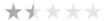

A taste explosion. Like, it literally feels as if someone put a grenade in your mouth and pulled the pin.

INGREDIENTS

1 (5-ounce / 142-g) can of tuna

3 tablespoons mayonnaise

5 ounces / 140 g rindless, seedless watermelon

METHOD

Open the can of tuna and drain off the brine or oil.

Put in a dish and add the mayo. Stir with a fork until it is thoroughly mixed in.

Put a ring mold onto a plate and put the mixture inside.

Cut the watermelon into bite-size shapes and place on top of the tuna-mayo mixture.

Remove the mold and enjoy.

SERVES 1

RUBBER BANDS

Tara, Canberra, Australia

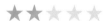

A bit like chewing gum. If they made chewing gum in terrible flavors.

INGREDIENT

1 pack of rubber bands

METHOD

Stretch 4–6 rubber bands around the plate and place the rest in the middle.

SERVES 0. WHAT WILL HAPPEN IF YOU EAT THESE? NO IDEA. PLEASE DON'T FIND OUT.

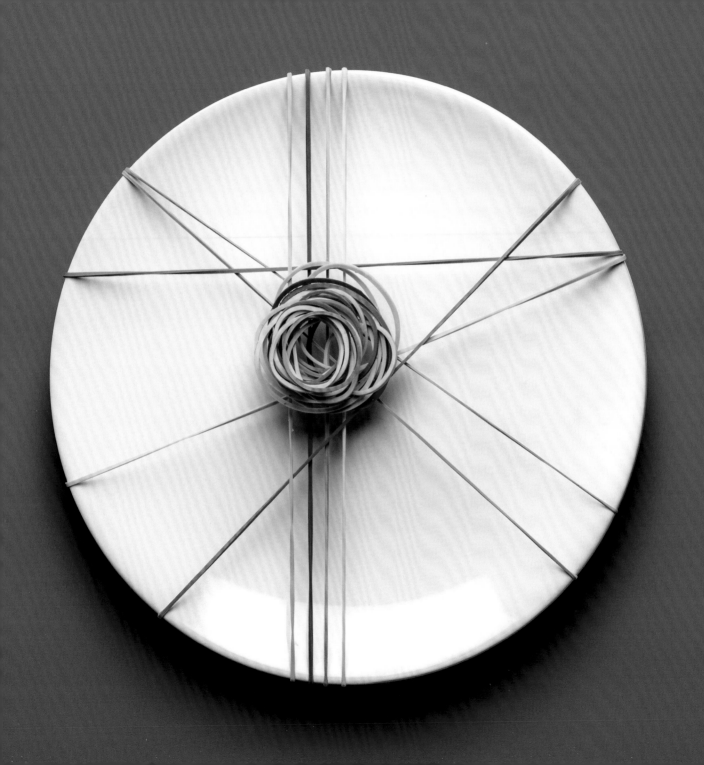

RUBBER BANDS

TARA, CANBERRA, AUSTRALIA

I'M NOT SURE HOW IT STARTED. I JUST STARTED TASTING RUBBER EVERYWHERE AND IN EVERYTHING. AND THEN I EVEN STARTED SMELLING IT. AFTER A WHILE I WANTED TO EAT IT, WHICH IS WHERE THE IDEA FOR THE RUBBER BANDS CAME FROM. I PREFERRED HOW THE THICK ONES TASTED—THEY HAD A STRONGER FLAVOR.

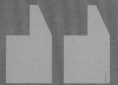

BACON AND MARS BAR BURGER

Suze, Hamburg, Germany

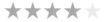

It's pretty crazy, but the good kind.
Not the one that runs after you in a mask with a chain saw.

INGREDIENTS

3 rashers of bacon

1 bread roll

Butter

2 Mars Bars

METHOD

Fry the bacon until it is crispy and then set aside.

Cut the bread roll in half and butter both sides generously.

Unwrap the Mars Bars and place them on the bottom half of the roll with the bacon on top.

Complete the burger with the top half of the bun and serve immediately.

_____

SERVES 1

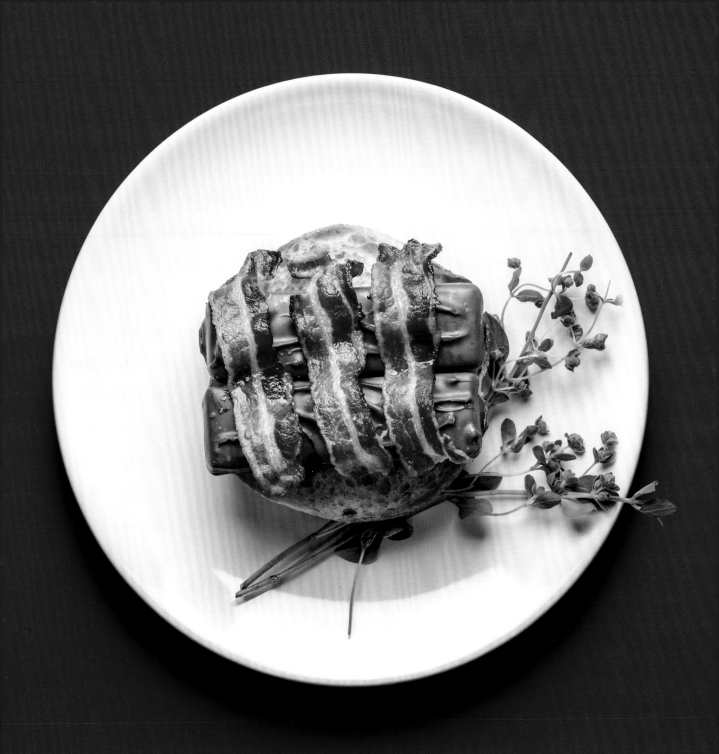

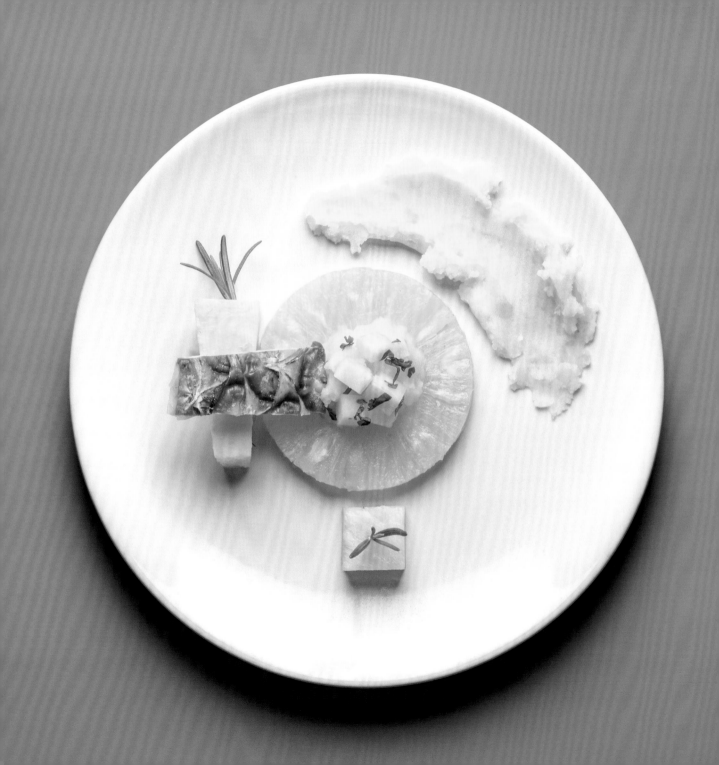

PINEAPPLE POTATOES

Julie, Johannesburg, South Africa

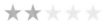

Some things just don't mix well—the Internet and productivity, hangovers and screaming toddlers, Legos and bare feet . . . add pineapples and potato to that list.

INGREDIENTS

1 teaspoon salt

2 medium potatoes

1 tablespoon butter

¼ cup / 60 ml milk

3 slices of pineapple

Rosemary and chopped chives, for garnish

METHOD

Boil a pot of water, adding the salt.

Peel the potatoes and cut them into quarters.

Boil the potatoes for about 15 minutes.

Drain.

Add the butter and milk and mash until smooth.

Add salt to taste.

Arrange the pineapple and mashed potato on a plate.

Garnish with rosemary and chives.

SERVES 1

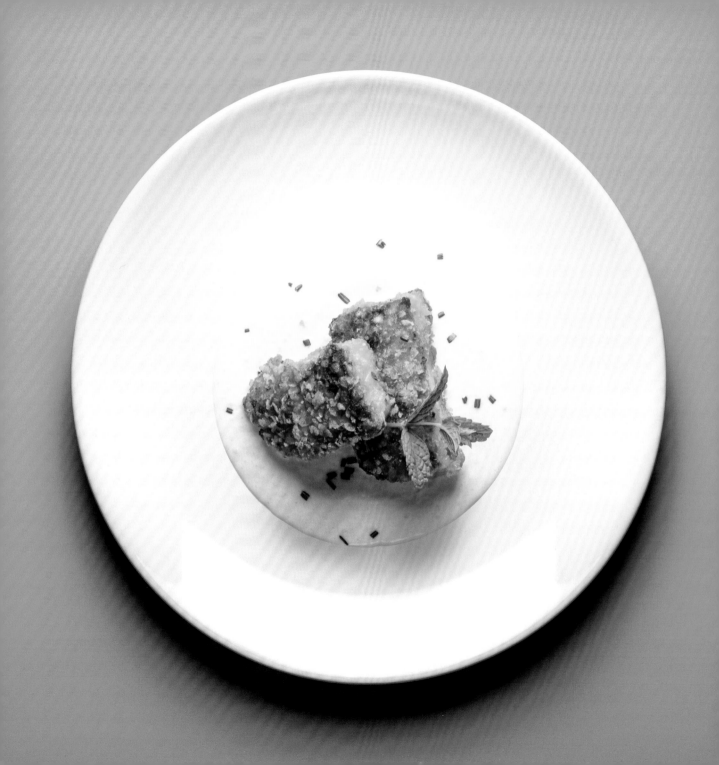

CHICKEN NUGGETS WITH WHIPPED CREAM

Jessica, North Adams, Massachusetts, USA

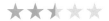

The flavor of whipped cream with the texture of a chicken nugget.
Somehow not as good as it sounds. We had to eat it. You don't.

INGREDIENTS

1 chicken breast

Salt

Pepper

1 egg

3 tablespoons bread crumbs

2 tablespoons all-purpose flour

Pinch of dried thyme

Pinch of dried basil

½ cup / 120 ml canola or sunflower oil

2 tablespoons heavy whipping cream (chilled)

1 teaspoon sugar

METHOD

Preheat the oven to 200°C / 400°F.

Cut the chicken into 2 x 1-inch (approx. 5 x 2.5-cm) rectangles and season with salt and pepper.

Set up three bowls: one with beaten egg, one with the bread crumbs, and one with the flour and spices mixed together.

Dip each piece of chicken first in the flour, then the egg, the bread crumbs.

Heat up the oil in a pan.

Fry the chicken about 7 minutes per side and set aside.

Beat the whipping cream in a bowl, gradually adding the sugar.

When it forms stiff peaks, it is ready.

Make a bed of whipped cream and place the chicken nuggets on top.

Watch in horror as the heat from the nuggets almost immediately melts the whipped cream back to its liquid form.

SERVES 1

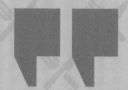

CHICKEN NUGGETS WITH WHIPPED CREAM

JESSICA, NORTH ADAMS, MASSACHUSETTS, USA

I craved a lot of saltiness and dairy during my pregnancy. I also ate banana splits every night. Sometimes I would put popcorn on my ice cream. I just happened to look in the fridge one day and see whipped cream and thought this would go great with fries. From there I would dip anything fried into whipped cream. Chicken nuggets, mozzarella sticks, mac and cheese bites, potato chips.

MY SON DOESN'T REALLY LIKE ANY FRIED FOODS, WHIPPED CREAM, CHOCOLATE SYRUP, ICE CREAM. I GUESS HE HAD ENOUGH DURING PREGNANCY. His teeth came early which I figured was due to all the calcium I consumed.

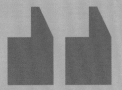

HOT FUDGE PIZZA

Shivawn, Chicago, USA

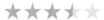

Kind of good in a bad way. Since chocolate and pizza are the two most addictive substances known to man, it's hard to stop eating. Be careful with this one.

INGREDIENTS

1 ham and olive pizza

¼ (14-ounce / 400-ml) can condensed milk

2 teaspoons cocoa powder (unsweetened)

1 tablespoon butter

⅛ teaspoon vanilla extract

METHOD

Remove your frozen pizza from the packaging and cook according to the instructions or order a ham and olive pizza from your local pizza restaurant. (Seriously, who makes a pizza from scratch?)

While you are waiting for your pizza, make the hot fudge sauce.

Pour the milk into a heavy saucepan and sift in the cocoa powder. Bring to a boil over medium heat while stirring often. Boil for 3 minutes while stirring constantly.

Remove the saucepan from the heat and add the butter. It should melt rapidly and can be stirred into the mixture.

Add the vanilla extract and stir.

Allow the hot fudge to cool until it is warm, but not hot enough to burn you.

Slice the pizza into twelve equal slices, if it is not already sliced.

Pour the hot fudge evenly over the entire pizza.

SERVES 1

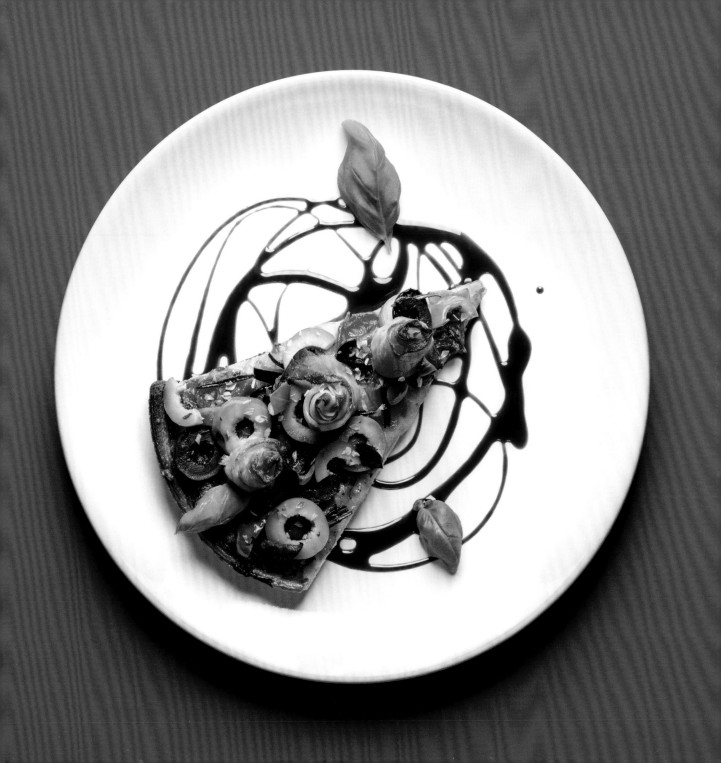

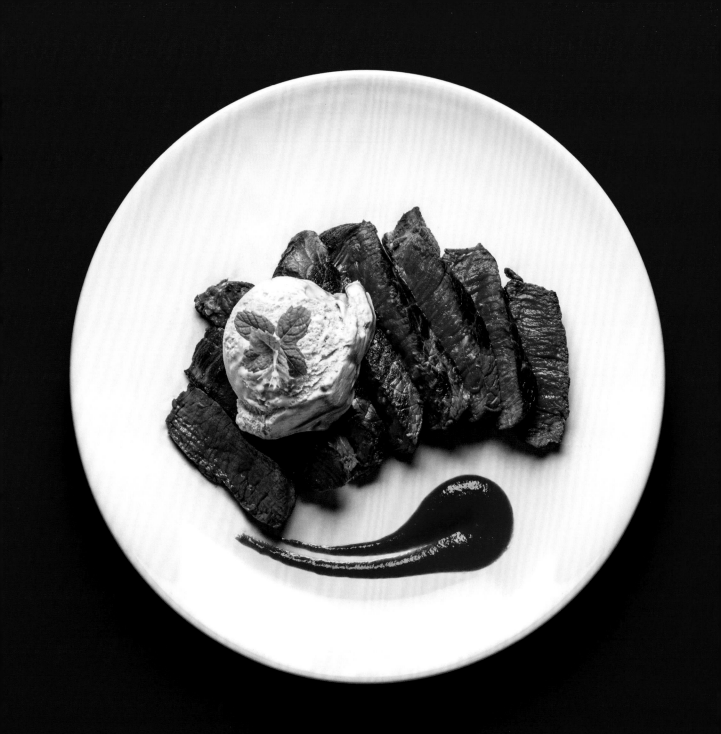

STEAK WITH ICE CREAM

Olivia, Greenville, South Carolina, USA

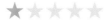

There is a special place in hell for people who ruin good steaks like this.
We'll save you a seat.

INGREDIENTS

3 tablespoons canola or sunflower oil

1 (7-ounce / 200-g) fillet steak

Salt

Pepper

1–2 scoops of ice cream (your choice of flavor)

METHOD

Heat the oil in a pan until hot.

Season the steak with salt and pepper. For a 1-inch / 2.5-cm-thick steak, fry for approximately 1½ minutes per side for rare, 2 minutes for medium, and 4–5 minutes for well done. If you are pregnant, sorry, but it's well done for you.

Remove the pan from the heat and let the steak rest at room temperature for about 5 minutes.

Add the ice cream on top and eat quickly before it melts.

SERVES 1

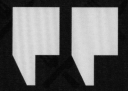

STEAK WITH ICE CREAM

OLIVIA, GREENVILLE, SOUTH CAROLINA, USA

I WAS CRAVING SOMETHING THAT WOULD FILL ME UP AND STEAK HAPPENED TO POP UP ON THE TV. BUT I DIDN'T WANT SOMETHING THAT WAS HOT, SO I PUT ICE CREAM ON TOP. I HAD TO HAVE IT AT LEAST ONCE A WEEK FOR ABOUT TWO MONTHS. THE FATHER OF MY CHILD THOUGHT IT WAS REVOLTING AND REFUSED TO WATCH ME EAT IT.

HAVING MY SON WAS THE BIGGEST BLESSING, BUT HE GAVE ME QUITE A FEW CRAZY CRAVINGS. I ALSO CRAVED HOT CHEETOS AND LUCKY CHARMS WITH MILK.

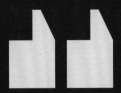

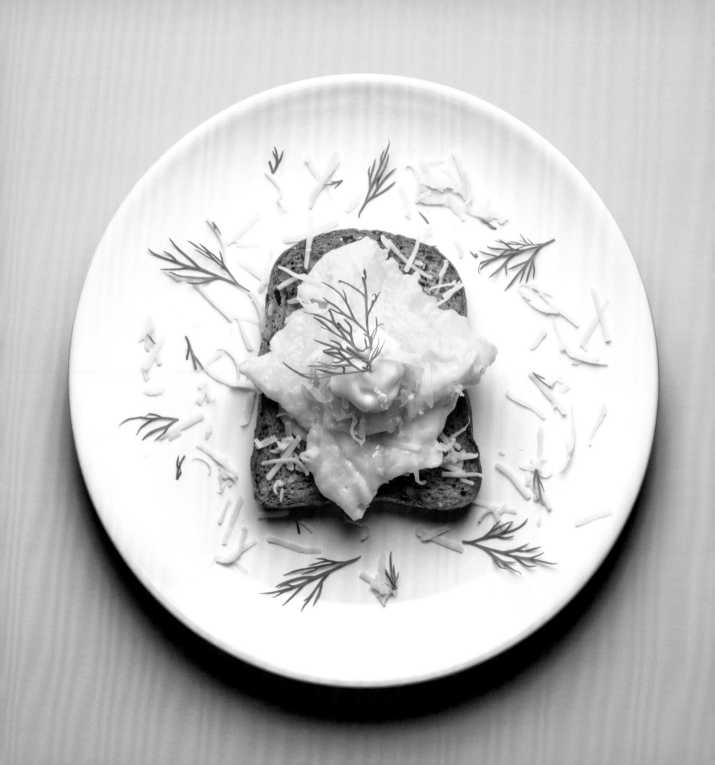

SCRAMBLED EGGS, CHEESE, AND SAUERKRAUT ON TOAST

Jerri, Westport, Connecticut, USA

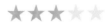

This is one dish we can wholeheartedly and unreservedly say is "It's all right, I guess."

INGREDIENTS

2 tablespoon butter

2 eggs

Salt

Pepper

¼ (14-ounce / 400-ml) can sauerkraut

Slice of brown bread

1 tablespoon mayonnaise

¼ cup / 40 g cheddar cheese

Fresh chopped dill, for garnish

METHOD

Melt the butter in a pan over medium heat.

Whisk the eggs in a bowl and add a pinch of salt and a grind or two of pepper for each egg.

Pour the egg mixture into the pan. After about 30 seconds, lift and fold with a spatula until it is cooked through.

Heat up the sauerkraut in the microwave.

Toast the bread and butter it.

Put the mayonnaise, scrambled egg, and sauerkraut on top of the bread, then sprinkle with cheese and garnish with dill.

SERVES 1

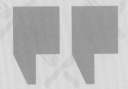

SCRAMBLED EGGS, CHEESE, AND SAUERKRAUT ON TOAST

JERRI, WESTPORT, CONNECTICUT, USA

I was living in Taiwan when I found out I was pregnant and all "American" foods made me nostalgic and long for home. From the get-go I wanted comfort food. One evening I was making a grilled cheese sandwich and some eggs. The idea of putting them together and adding sauerkraut just sounded heavenly. From the first bite, I was totally hooked. The tang of the sauerkraut mixed with the creaminess of the cheese was oddly satisfying.

My cravings were all about this combination of eggs, cheese, and sauerkraut when I was pregnant. I would use about a quarter of a can of sauerkraut on each sandwich, so there was a lot of vinegar flavor coming through. Luckily my partner was Scottish and grew up eating haggis so he wasn't fazed in the slightest by it.

I ATE THIS SANDWICH EVERY EVENING FOR ABOUT SEVEN MONTHS. IT BECAME A RITUAL. I CAN'T STAND SAUERKRAUT NOW.

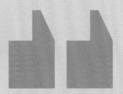

DOG FOOD

Elizabeth, San Antonio, Texas, USA

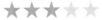

*Dogs love their food. But dogs also eat their own puke, so there
was a fair amount of dread before trying this one. Surprisingly, it was very bland.
Like a regular cracker with a hint of a taste of beef broth.
Good for us, but maybe not so good for dogs?*

INGREDIENTS

1½ ounces / 40 g dry dog food

METHOD

Pick out the pieces that most appeal to you and arrange
them on a plate.

SERVES 0 PEOPLE. 1 DOG.

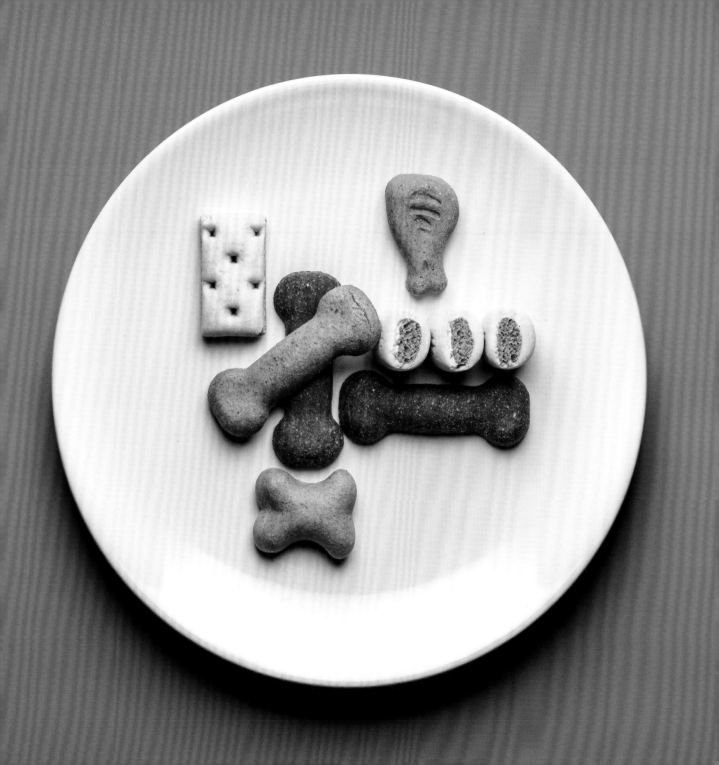

DOG
FOOD

ELIZABETH, SAN ANTONIO, TEXAS, USA

I was feeding my dog one day and the dog food smelled great. When I first tasted it, it was sort of one of those "awww" moments when you eat something you have been wanting for a really long time. After I had my son I tried it again and let's just say I definitely wasn't pregnant anymore! I don't know what I was thinking. BACK THEN I WOULD GET A ZIPLOCK BAG AND TAKE THE PIECES I WANTED TO EAT, SO I COULD HAVE IT ANYTIME "ON THE GO."

My whole family thought it was disgusting; my mom even bought a different brand to discourage me from eating it. I was pretty mad. My parents would say, "Your baby is gonna come out acting like a dog with all that dog food you're eating." Then when my son was about two, maybe almost three, I caught him in the kitchen sitting next to the dog bowl eating dog food. Safe to say he didn't like it, but you live and you learn.

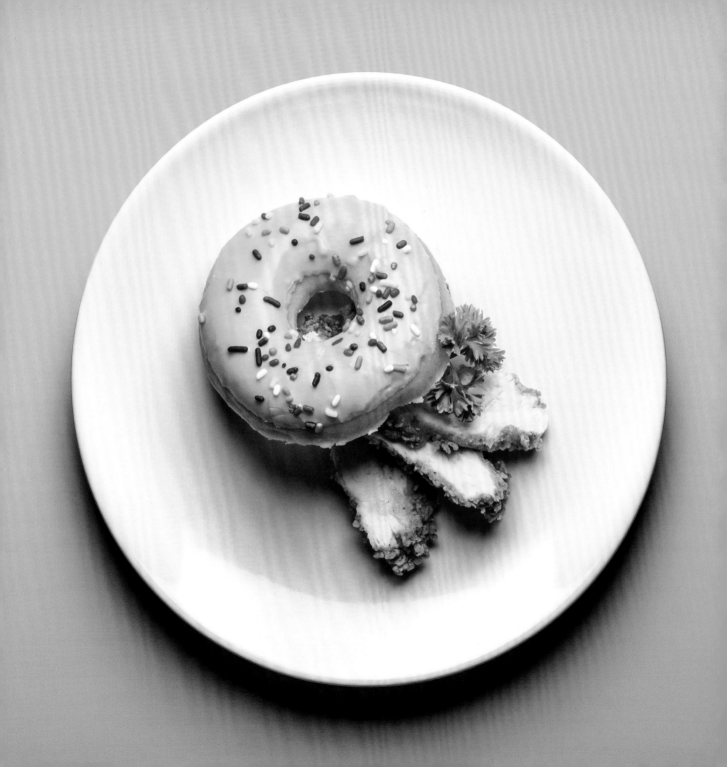

FRIED CHICKEN DONUT BURGER

Kristina, Tallahassee, Florida, USA

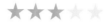

Sadly, the satisfaction-to-calories ratio just isn't high enough.

FRIED CHICKEN

Vegetable oil for deep frying

¼ cup / 30 g all-purpose flour

Pinch of paprika

Pinch of garlic salt

Pinch of cayenne pepper

Pinch of onion powder

Pinch of salt

Pinch of white pepper

1 chicken breast

2 tablespoons buttermilk

METHOD

Heat the oil in a deep fryer or large iron skillet to 325ºF / 160ºC.

Put the flour and spices in a resealable plastic bag and shake to mix.

Coat the chicken in the buttermilk and then put it into the bag with the seasoned flour and shake well.

Deep fry the chicken breast for about 10 minutes.

Remove from the oil and let cool on a rack.

Refry the chicken until crispy. Remove and drain on a rack.

(recipe continues)

DONUTS

¼ ounce / 7 g active dry yeast

2 teaspoons sugar

2 teaspoons warm water
(100°F / 40–45°C)

2 tablespoons warm milk

1 teaspoon butter

½ cup / 60 g all-purpose flour

⅛ teaspoon baking soda

Light pinch of salt

¼ of a beaten egg

3 tablespoons confectioners' sugar

½ teaspoon warm water

Red food coloring

Sprinkles

To make the donut, first put the yeast and sugar in the warm water. Stir and let sit for 5 minutes.

Heat the milk and butter in the microwave until it just starts to boil.

Put half the flour with the baking soda and salt into a mixing bowl.

Pour the egg into the mixing bowl along with the yeast mixture and milk.

Mix until smooth, slowly adding the rest of the flour until you have a dough-like texture that doesn't stick to the sides of the bowl.

Cover the bowl and put it in a warm place for 1 hour or until it has doubled in size.

Form into a donut shape and deep fry in the same oil you used for the chicken.

Cook until light golden brown on both sides, turning once.

Set aside on a paper towel while you make the glaze.

Mix the confectioners' sugar, ½ teaspoon warm water, and a little red food coloring together. Be careful not to put in too much food coloring, just a tiny amount will get the pink color you are looking for.

Pour over the warm donut. Add the sprinkles while the glaze is still wet.

Allow the donut to cool and the glaze to set.

Cut the donut in half as you would a bread roll.

Place the fried chicken inside as you would a burger. You can place the breast whole or slice it up first.

Serve.

ALTERNATIVE METHOD

Turn twenty-one steps into two steps by simply buying a donut and piece of fried chicken. We won't judge you. Promise.

SERVES 1

COAL

Amanda, São Paulo, Brazil

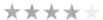

Surprisingly, it tasted like nothing. Slightly gritty nothing. It gets 4 stars because the relief that it wasn't terrible was absolutely delicious.

INGREDIENTS

Coal

METHOD

Put a piece of coal on a plate.

SERVES 0. SHOULD YOU EAT THIS?
A BIG NO WITH A SIDE OF NOPE.

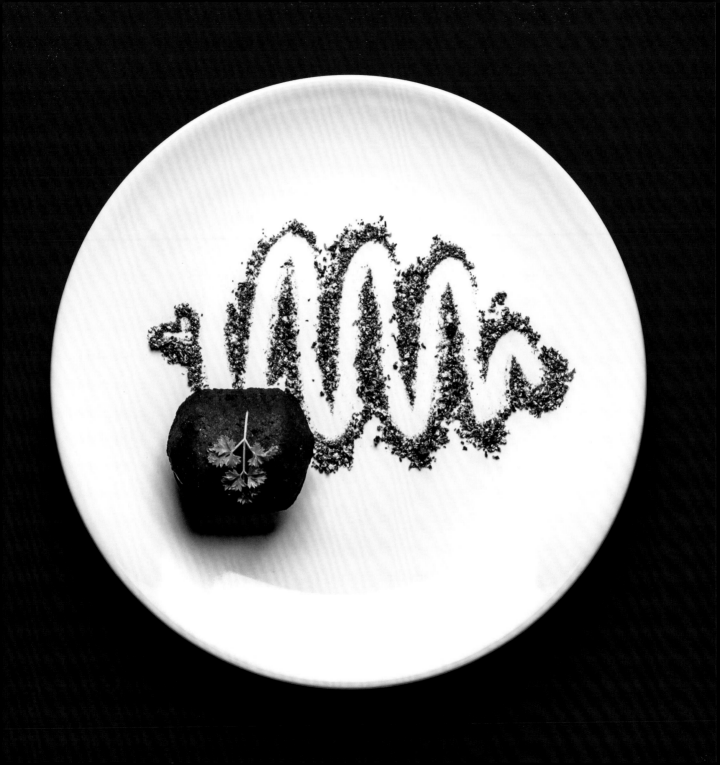

CHICKEN WITH FROSTING

Rachel, West Valley City, Utah, USA

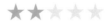

It's that couple you know from the second they get together that it's all going to end in tears.

INGREDIENTS

2 tablespoons butter

1 cup / 110 g confectioners' sugar

⅓ teaspoon milk

Food coloring, e.g., yellow, blue, and pink, or your preference

Salt

Pepper

1 chicken breast

2 tablespoons olive oil

Maraschino cherry, for garnish

METHOD

Blend the butter and sugar together in a bowl with a spoon or mixer until well mixed.

Stir in the milk.

Separate the frosting into portions and add a different-colored food coloring to each one. Mix each thoroughly until the color is uniform.

Put in the fridge to chill until the chicken is ready.

Sprinkle salt and pepper on both sides of the chicken breast.

Heat olive oil in a pan to medium heat.

Fry the chicken for 10–12 minutes, turning occasionally to ensure even cooking. If the chicken is cooking too fast or getting charred on the outside, turn down the heat. When the chicken is cooked through and the juices run clear, it is ready.

Remove the pan from the heat and slice the chicken into slightly angled slices.

Add the frosting on or around the chicken in a decorative pattern.

Place the cherry strategically on the frosting to garnish.

Serve.

SERVES 1

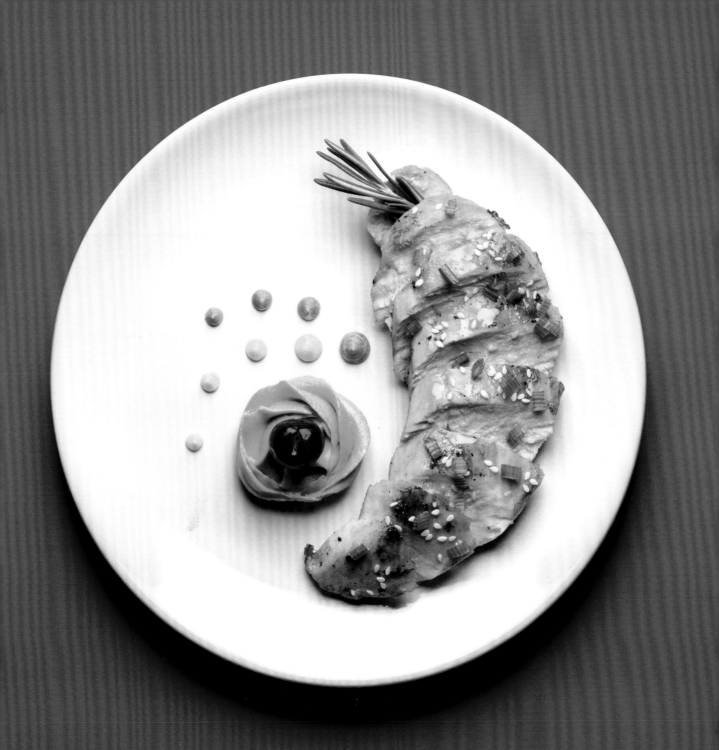

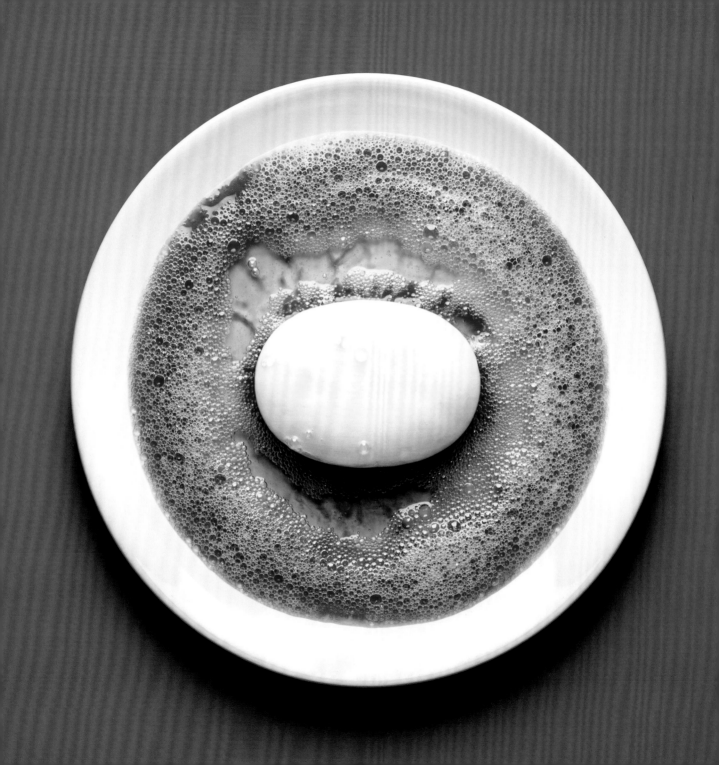

MEDLEY OF SOAPS

Jannel, Hexham, Northumberland, England

★ ★ ★ ★ ★

*Do not try this. Ever. Ignoring this warning isn't like ignoring
the expiration date on a yogurt. It's like ignoring the warning of the lifeguard on
the beach who tells you not to enter the shark-infested waters.*

INGREDIENTS

*Liquid hand soap for
sauce / decoration*

1 bar of soap

METHOD

Put a squirt of the hand soap aside; mix it vigorously with a little water until it forms foam.

Use different-colored liquid hand soaps and foam to create delicious-looking patterns.

Finish the dish with a bar of soap in the middle.

SERVES 0—IF IN DOUBT ABOUT WHETHER YOU SHOULD EAT THIS, REFER TO THE REVIEW AT THE TOP OF THE PAGE.

MEDLEY
OF SOAPS

JANNEL, HEXHAM, NORTHUMBERLAND, ENGLAND

I have always loved the smell of soap like a lot of people do, but during each of my four pregnancies I was overcome with the urge to lick or bite bars of soap. ALTHOUGH THE TASTE OF IT WOULD MAKE ME COUGH AFTER A WHILE AND COULD GET QUITE OVERPOWERING, I JUST COULDN'T STOP. There were a few times I would grate the soap like cheese and nibble it, even putting it on toast or crackers like a topping. I would say I ate it at least three times a week, not too often as it caused heartburn after too much. Most other people thought I was totally nuts except other women who had also experienced the same craving. There have been times even when I'm not pregnant that I will randomly have a sneaky lick of a bar of soap but generally the urge just strikes during pregnancy.

CUSTARD, JELLY, PEANUT BUTTER, BANANA, AND CREAM SANDWICH

Gemma, Ballarat, Victoria, Australia

The genius is it's actually a cake but you get to call it a sandwich, which totally makes it suitable for lunch, dinner, breakfast, in-between snacks . . . now.

INGREDIENTS

2 slices of white bread

⅓ banana

1½ tablespoons peanut butter

1 tablespoon jelly

1 tablespoon custard

Whipped cream

METHOD

Toast the bread

Slice the banana into equal slices.

Add the peanut butter, banana, jelly, and custard in layers to one slice of bread.

Put the second piece of bread on top and finish with whipped cream.

Cut diagonally across and serve.

SERVES 1

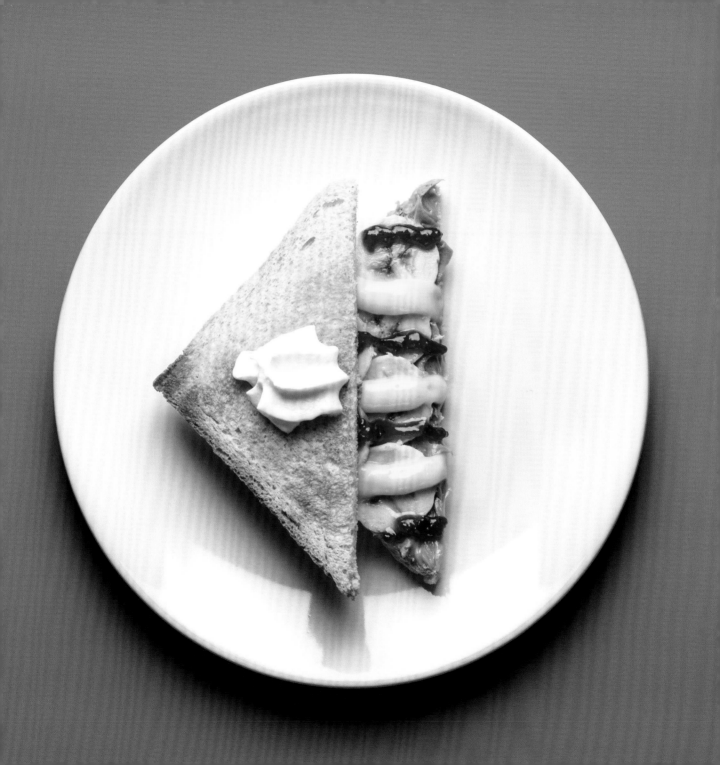

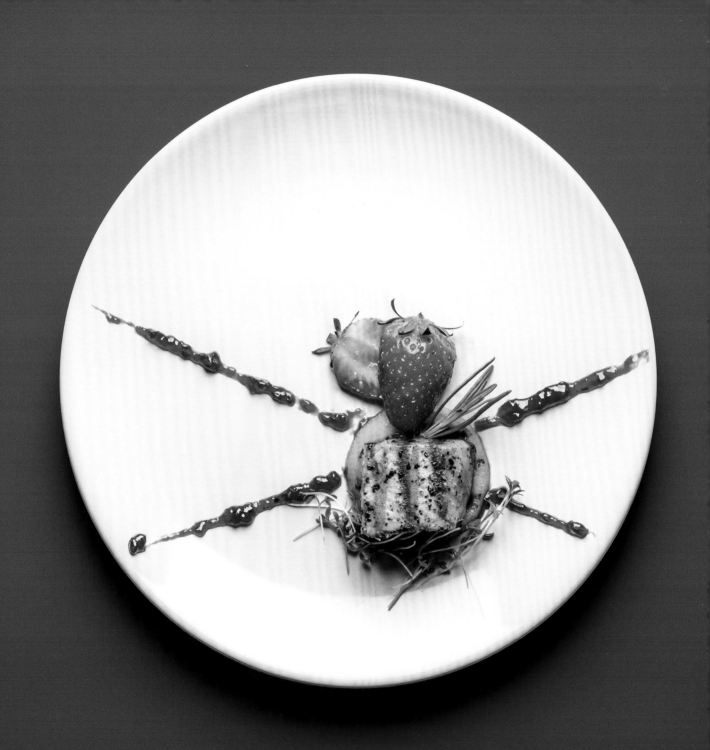

TUNA WITH STRAWBERRY JAM

Sarah, Norwich, East Anglia, England

It's kind of like that time your mom got a bit experimental in the kitchen and served up something "new" she just "wanted to try." It's not going to kill you, but you might just end up feeding most of it to the dog.

INGREDIENTS

2 tablespoons olive oil

Salt

Pepper

*1 tuna steak, approximately
4 ounces / 100 g*

2 tablespoons strawberry jam

Several slices of lemon

1 strawberry, halved, for garnish

*Rosemary and sprouts, for garnish
if desired*

METHOD

Heat the oil on high heat.

Salt and pepper the tuna steak, then fry for about 5 minutes per side.

Remove the steak from the heat and cut into squares about 2.5 x 2.5 inches / 6 x 6 cm in size.

Place each square on a slice of lemon and arrange approximately 1 teaspoon of jam on the plate in stripes, with garnish as desired.

Eat the square with the jam as sauce and repeat until full.

SERVES 1

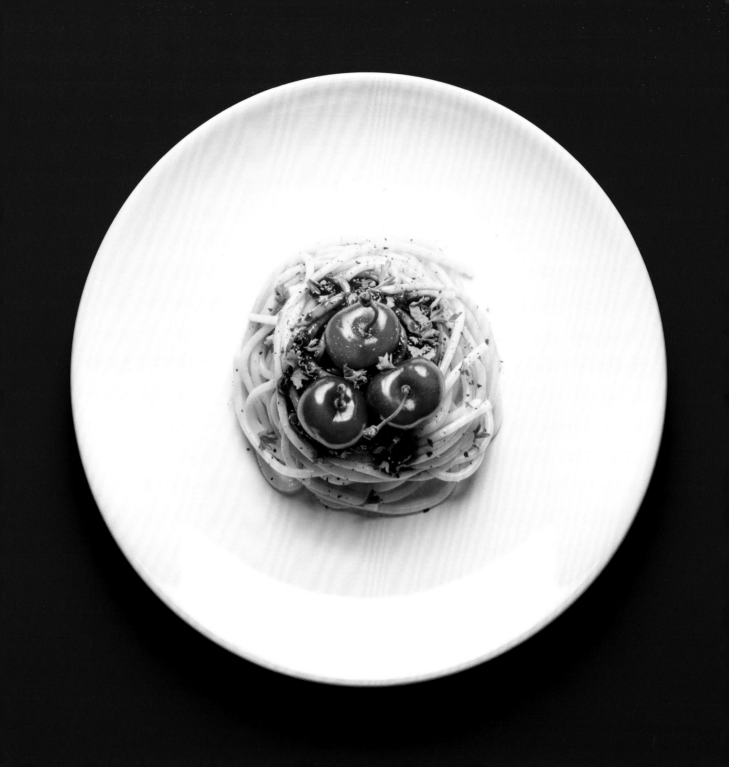

CHERRY SPAGHETTI

Leanne, Penticton, British Columbia, Canada

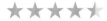

Religions have been founded on less divine experiences than this.

INGREDIENTS

1½ cups / 340 g fresh cherries, pitted and stems removed

1¼ tablespoons sugar

1 tablespoon butter

3 tablespoons water

1 tablespoon cornstarch

1 teaspoon salt

2 ounces / 70 g spaghetti

METHOD

Add 1 cup / 225 g cherries to a pot with the sugar, butter, and 1 tablespoon of water and bring to a boil on medium heat.

Simmer for 3 minutes on a lower heat.

In a separate bowl mix the cornstarch with 2 tablespoons of water until smooth.

Slowly pour the cornstarch mixture into the cherry mixture, stirring constantly.

Simmer while stirring for about 3 minutes, then remove the pot from the heat.

Bring a pot of water to a boil, adding the salt.

Add the spaghetti and cook for about 10 minutes or follow the cooking instructions on the box, stirring occasionally to prevent clumping.

Drain the pasta.

Pour on the sauce and stir in the remaining fresh cherries.

Serve.

_____

SERVES 1

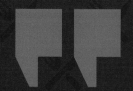

CHERRY
SPAGHETTI

LEANNE, PENTICTON, BRITISH COLUMBIA, CANADA

I COULDN'T DECIDE IF I WANTED SPAGHETTI OR CHERRIES. SO I DECIDED TO MIX THE CHERRIES WITH THE SPAGHETTI. IT WAS LOVE AT FIRST BITE. MY HUSBAND THOUGHT IT WAS STRANGE. FIVE YEARS LATER AND HE WILL STILL MENTION IT EVERY TIME WE HAVE SPAGHETTI.

PICKLED PIG'S FOOT
WITH CORNFLAKES AND MILK

Vivian, Tucson, Arizona, USA

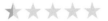

Gloopy, fatty, vinegary milk and a mutilated foot in a cereal bowl.
This is a valid alternative to the death penalty.

INGREDIENTS

1 pickled pig's foot

1¼ cups / 300 ml milk

1 ounce / 30 g frosted cornflakes

METHOD

Place the pig's foot in a bowl.

Add the milk and cornflakes.

Serve.

SERVES 1 UNFORTUNATE SOUL

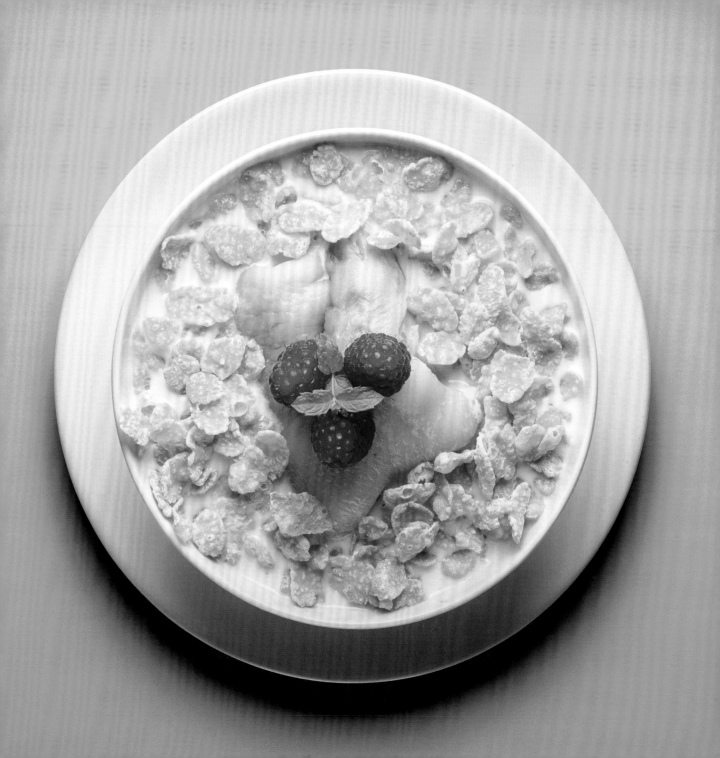

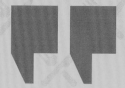

PICKLED PIG'S FOOT WITH CORNFLAKES AND MILK

VIVIAN, TUCSON, ARIZONA, USA

Thirty-three years ago, when I was pregnant with my second child, I had a very specific craving. I would get a large bowl, place a pig's foot in it, then pour frosted flakes on top and fill the bowl with milk. First, I would eat the cereal and milk, leaving the pig's foot for last. The coolness of the milk felt good in my tummy and the sweet/sour fulfilled my craving. Couldn't get enough for nine months. It was so good. I ate it—no kidding—at least twice a day and late at night. My husband at the time couldn't keep the cereal or pig's feet in stock. **ONCE IN THE MIDDLE OF THE NIGHT I HAD NO PIG'S FEET. I WOKE UP MY HUSBAND AND HE WAS SO UPSET THAT I WAS UPSET—ALL THE STORES WERE CLOSED. SO HE WENT BAR HOPPING AND BOUGHT ALL THE HUGE JARS OF PIG FEET! THAT LASTED ME A COUPLE OF MONTHS.**

I've often wondered if the crazy cravings helped produce the wonderful people I call my children. Smart, loving, caring, intelligent human beings and good looking, too! I know this did not come from me . . . had to be the cravings!

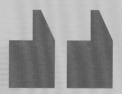

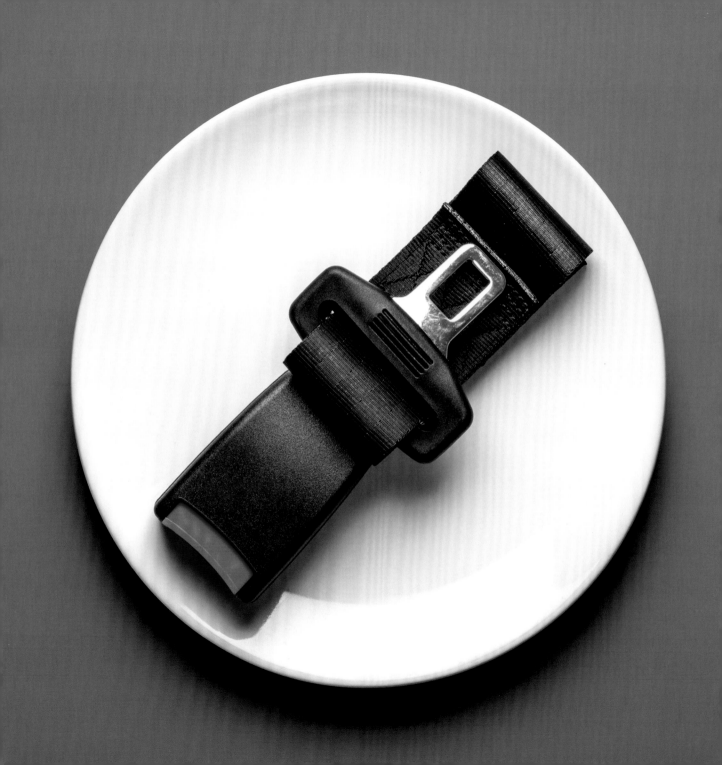

SEAT BELT

Patricia, Addison, Alabama, USA

*Seat belts were first invented by the Englishman George Cayley
in the mid-nineteenth century. Since then, they have been used to help keep people
safer in accidents. And after tasting them, it is clear that this should
continue to be their only purpose. Forever.*

INGREDIENTS

1 seat belt

METHOD

This can be enjoyed "raw" in the car by simply chewing on an available seat belt. Or you can remove a seat belt and gnaw on it in the comfort of your own home.

SERVES 0. DO YOURSELF, YOUR TEETH, AND YOUR DIGESTIVE SYSTEM A FAVOR AND DON'T EAT THIS.

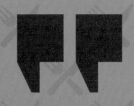

SEAT BELT

PATRICIA, ADDISON, ALABAMA, USA

It was my first pregnancy, and a few months after I found out I caught myself chewing on seat belts—my car, someone else's car, it didn't matter. I would start chewing on them without even realizing it. It happened pretty much every time I got in a car. I would try not to, I mean, who eats someone's seat belt? But it didn't matter; within a few minutes I would be chewing on it. I got a lot of crazy looks over that! My friends and family just laughed at me, they thought it was gross, but hilarious at the same time. After a while, it got to the point that it was concerning enough to actually talk with the doctor about it. **HE JUST SMILED AT ME WITH A LOOK OF PITY IN HIS EYES AND SAID THAT I WAS ACTUALLY CRAVING THE SALT IN THE SEAT BELT FROM PEOPLE'S SWEAT.** Although I was probably unaware of it, I could smell it because my senses were enhanced from pregnancy, and that is why I chewed on them. He said not to worry, though, other pregnant women had done the same thing. And suggested wrapping a hand towel around the seatbelt to fix the problem. It did, thankfully. I never ate another seat belt after that. I did try adding extra salt to other things to satisfy the craving, but it just wasn't the same as a sweaty seatbelt.

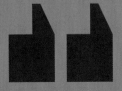

SARDINES, MUSTARD, AND COFFEE

Stephanie, Southaven, Mississippi, USA

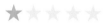

The three different flavors are like a trio of punches in the gut ending with a particularly brutal sardine uppercut.

INGREDIENTS

2 sardines

1 teaspoon olive oil

Squeeze of lemon juice

Salt

4 tablespoons boiled water

1 heaped teaspoon Dijon mustard

1 teaspoon instant coffee

METHOD

Heat the oven to 350°F / 180°C.

Gut, wash, and descale the sardines if it has not already been done.

Brush with olive oil, sprinkle with lemon juice, and season with salt.

Bake for 10 minutes.

Boil the water.

Place the Dijon mustard on the plate and place the sardines on top.

Stir the coffee into the boiling water and use as a sauce with the sardines.

Serve.

SERVES 1

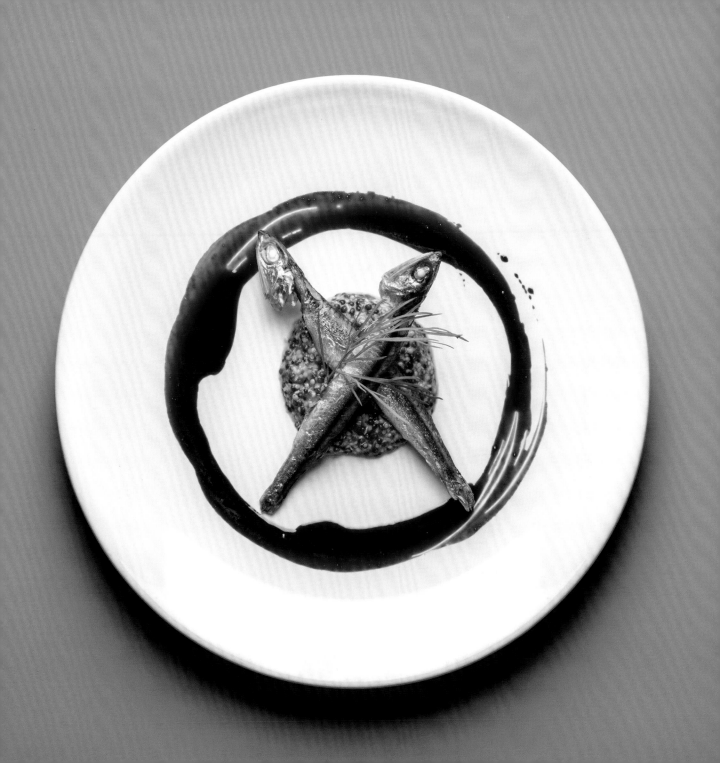

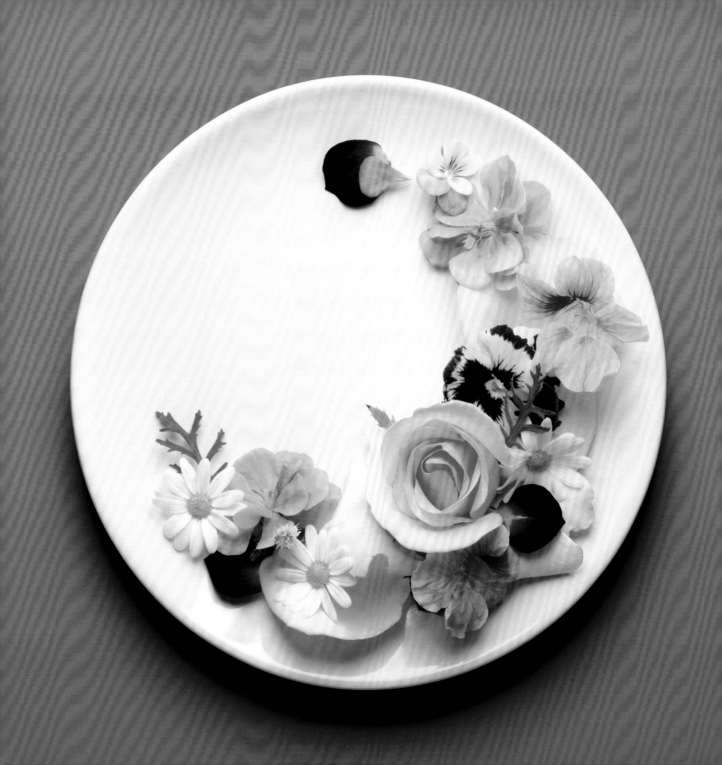

FLOWER SALAD

Trisha, Pinckney, Michigan, USA

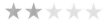

It's the kind of thing you'll really appreciate if you end up alone, stranded in the wild. Like knowing which beetles are a good source of protein or how to fashion a rope from your own hair. Unfortunately, that's probably the only scenario in which you will really appreciate it.

INGREDIENTS

Any edible flowers that are in season can be added to this salad. Make sure the plants have been grown in a way that is suitable for human consumption, i.e., no harmful pesticides or fertilizers.

For this salad, we used:
Roses
Pansies
Daisies
Mint flowers
Nasturtium
Pineapple sage

METHOD

Mix around two handfuls of different flowers and petals together. Add a rose to the side of the plate and then scatter the rest of the flowers in a semicircle around it for an aesthetically pleasing effect.

Enjoy.

SERVES 1

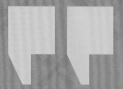

FLOWER
SALAD

TRISHA, PINCKNEY, MICHIGAN, USA

I wanted to eat flowers during my first pregnancy. MY HUSBAND BROUGHT ME HOME SOME ROSES AND I HAD TO FIGHT THE URGE TO CHOMP THE HEADS OF THEM LIKE A BILLY GOAT. I panicked and immediately looked online for symptoms of pica (first-time mom, I googled something every 10 minutes) and didn't see anything for flower cravings; instead I was pleased to find that not only is there an extensive list of edible flowers but that some are quite a delicacy! I went straight to my garden and plucked a few from my borage and tomato plants to taste-test and managed to keep the roses in a pretty vase.

I discovered borage flowers taste like cucumber and I would munch on other local flowers like honeysuckle and clover. It didn't seem to matter which flowers I ate to satisfy my cravings—I simply wanted to eat flowers. My husband started to tease me about eating things from the yard and my friends (many of whom had yet to become pregnant) laughed it off as completely bizarre, as did I.

I actually do still eat flowers. Now they have many lilac flower recipes and when I see those I get sad that I didn't know about those back then! I grew up in the country where foraging the occasional mushrooms, asparagus, or other local wild delicacies was normal and I simply added flowers to my knowledge base. They've been part of our lives ever since. Just the other day my four-year-old daughter and I sat in the yard and taste-tested clovers. My girls will pick something and bring it indoors and say, "Momma, look what I brought for you! Can we eat them?" For the record there is a huge amount of edible flowers out there! Obviously we refrain from anything possibly treated with chemicals but anything else is fair game.

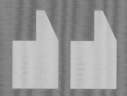

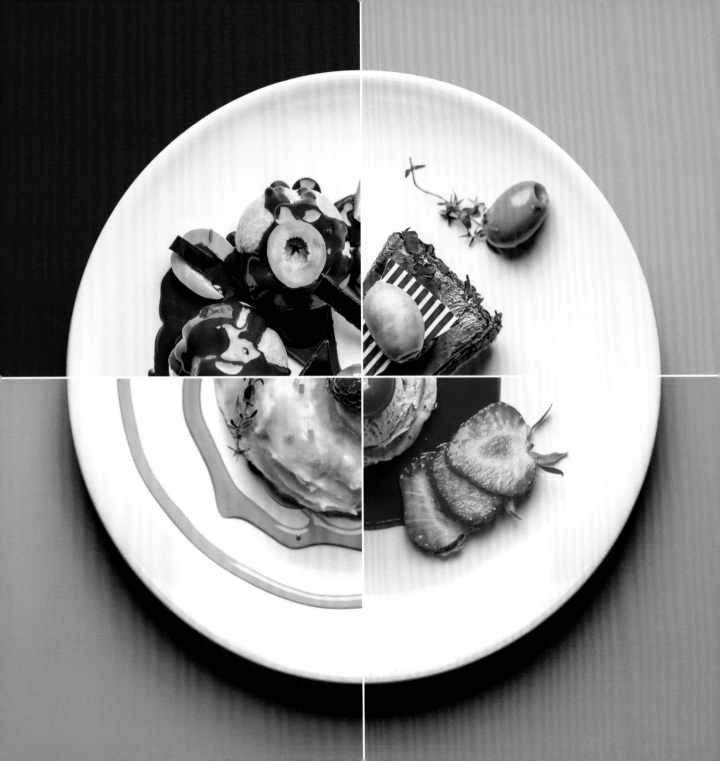

DESSERT

When your belly is already huge, but you aren't quite done yet. That is the third trimester. Or dessert time. Or both. In this chapter a few surprise ingredients turn all types of classic desserts on their head.

Discover the smoothie of your nightmares, the first dessert with shrimp in it, and one of the world's best-kept secrets: that you don't have to be pregnant to enjoy Pickles and Ice Cream. In fact, you don't even have to be hungry.

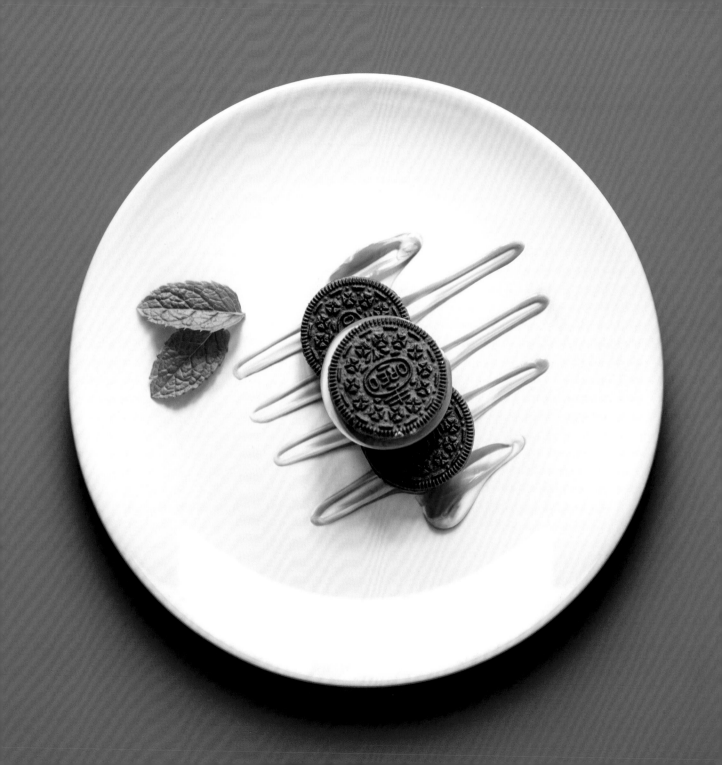

TOOTHPASTE COOKIES

Flavia, Goiânia, Goiás, Brazil

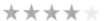

*The only thing better than chocolate and mint together is having
a cookie that brushes your teeth for you.*

INGREDIENTS

3 Oreos

1 tube of toothpaste

METHOD

Twist the Oreos to separate them.

Put a generous layer of toothpaste on top of the filling and then put the Oreo back together.

SERVES 0—THERE IS A REASON YOU ALWAYS SPIT TOOTHPASTE OUT. PLEASE MAKE SURE YOU CONTINUE THAT HABIT HERE.

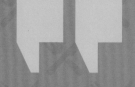

TOOTHPASTE OREOS

FLAVIA, GOIÂNIA, GOIÁS, BRAZIL

I was already seven months pregnant when I discovered this wonder, so I only had it about four or five times. It was actually really tasty and I even had a favorite brand of toothpaste. I got the idea when I saw my cousin eating an Oreo with whipped cream, which reminded me a lot of toothpaste. The thought seemed a bit crazy, though, so I tried to just forget about it. But then, three days later, I was at home, bored and dying of heartburn and just couldn't resist. When I tried it: poof! My heartburn went away as if by magic.

THE ONLY ONE WHO CAUGHT ME EATING IT WAS MY MOTHER. BUT SHE DIDN'T JUDGE ME BECAUSE SHE HAD EATEN A LOT OF LIQUID SOAP DURING HER PREGNANCY. She tasted the Toothpaste Oreos, too, but she hated them. I tried it again about nine months after I gave birth. But when I wasn't pregnant it was horrible.

My kids actually love Oreos. And toothpaste, too. They ask me to brush their teeth all the time. But they never tried the two together— at least not to my knowledge.

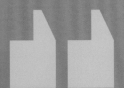

ICE CREAM AND CHILE SAUCE

Eunice, Roseburg, Oregon, USA

....

★ ★ ★ ★ ★

Horrible.

....

INGREDIENTS

2 scoops of ice cream

Sweet chile sauce / hot sauce

METHOD

Scoop ice cream into a dish.

Pour the chile sauce over it.

————————

SERVES 1

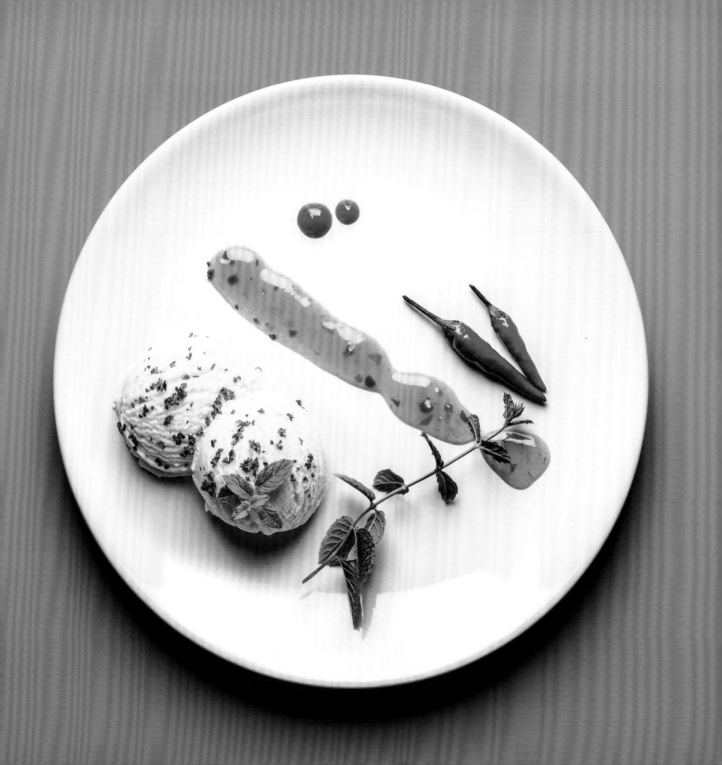

BEAN AND CREAM DREAM

Sandra, Zürich, Switzerland

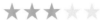

Try it. Shrug. Continue with your life.

INGREDIENTS

1 teaspoon salt

2 ounces / 50 g green beans

1 tablespoon butter

1 can whipped cream

METHOD

Fill a saucepan with water, add the salt, and bring to a boil.

Blanch the beans for about 4 minutes, then remove the saucepan from the heat and drain.

Sauté the beans in melted butter over medium heat.

Spray whipped cream onto a plate in the most artistic shape you are capable of and arrange the beans around it. Eat as you would chips and dip.

SERVES 1

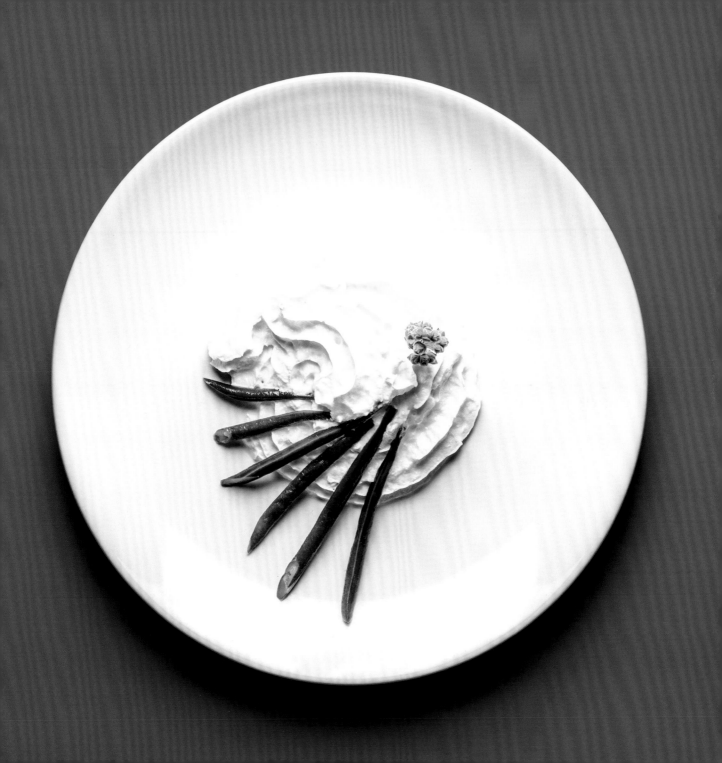

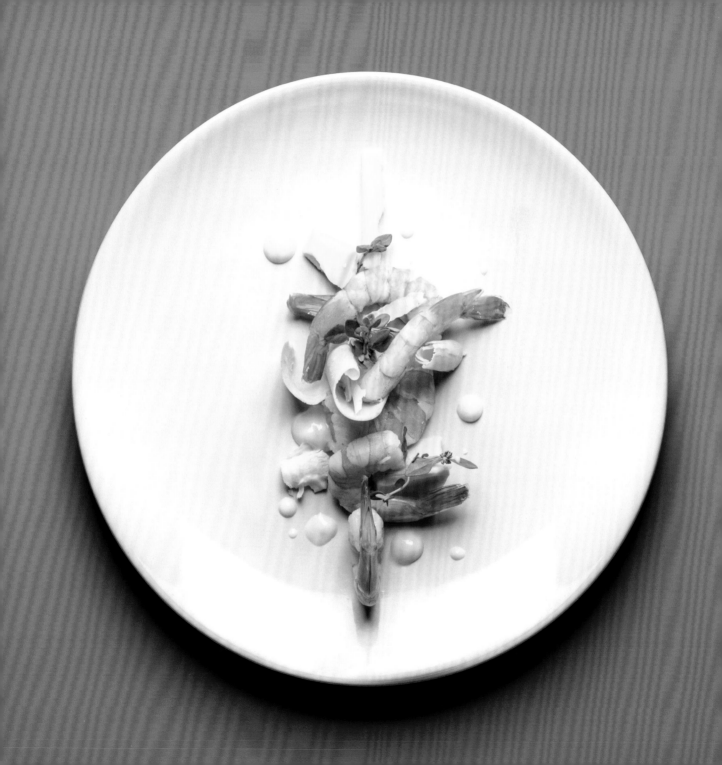

SHRIMP WITH WHITE CHOCOLATE

Donna, Midwest City, Oklahoma, USA

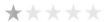

Sweet and shrimpy fight to the death—possibly yours.

INGREDIENTS

*2 ounces / Approx. 60 g
white chocolate*

*2 ounces / Approx 60 g cooked,
shelled, and deveined shrimp*

METHOD

Melt half the white chocolate over boiling water in
a metal bowl or heatproof glass bowl. Make sure the bowl
is not touching the water.

Dip each shrimp halfway into the chocolate and then
refrigerate for an hour.

You may also want to make some white chocolate
drops for decoration.

When the chocolate is hard, serve on a plate.

Garnish with shavings of the remaining white chocolate.

SERVES 1

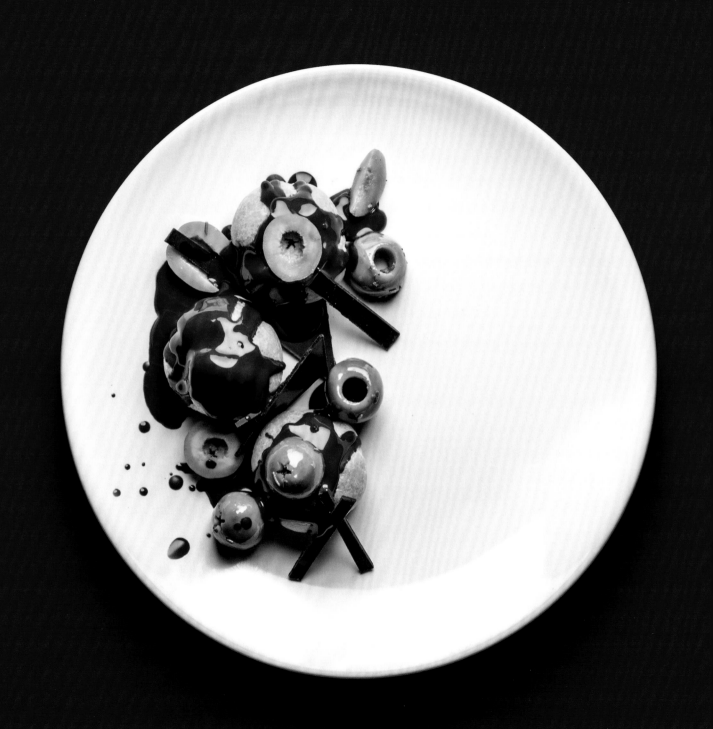

PROFITEROLES AND OLIVES

Andreea, London, England

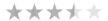

Depending on how much olive you have, it can give the profiterole an interesting salty edge or karate chop the flavor into oblivion.

INGREDIENTS

⅓ cup / 78 ml water

2 tablespoons and 2 teaspoons butter

Pinch of salt

⅓ cup / 40 g all-purpose flour

1 egg

⅓ cup / 78 ml heavy cream

1 tablespoon confectioners' sugar

3 ounces / 85 g chocolate

6 green olives, roughly chopped

METHOD

Preheat the oven to 425°F / 220°C.

Boil the water, butter, and salt in a pan.

Remove the pan from the heat and sift in the flour, stirring continuously and vigorously until the mixture is smooth. Mix in the eggs when the mixture is cool.

On a baking tray lined with baking paper, arrange 1-inch / 2½-cm circles of the mixture.

Bake for 20–25 minutes or until puffed up and golden brown.

Allow the pastries to cool.

Beat the cream and sugar together until the cream forms soft peaks.

Poke a small hole in the bottom of the pastries and pipe the whipped cream inside.

Melt the chocolate in a heat-proof glass bowl over boiling water.

As soon as the chocolate is melted, pour over the pastries.

Sprinkle the olives over the profiteroles.

SERVES 1

BEEF JERKY AND SKITTLES

Monica, Fort Worth, Texas, USA

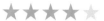

*Since they are both chewy it just tastes like beef jerky with
an extra, secret seasoning. Except it's not a secret. It's Skittles. Spread the word.*

INGREDIENTS

5 purple Skittles

5 green Skittles

5 yellow Skittles

5 orange Skittles

5 red Skittles

½ ounce / 15 g beef jerky

METHOD

Arrange the Skittles in lines of color like a rainbow.

Place the beef jerky next to it.

Make sure to eat one or two Skittles with every piece of jerky.

SERVES 1

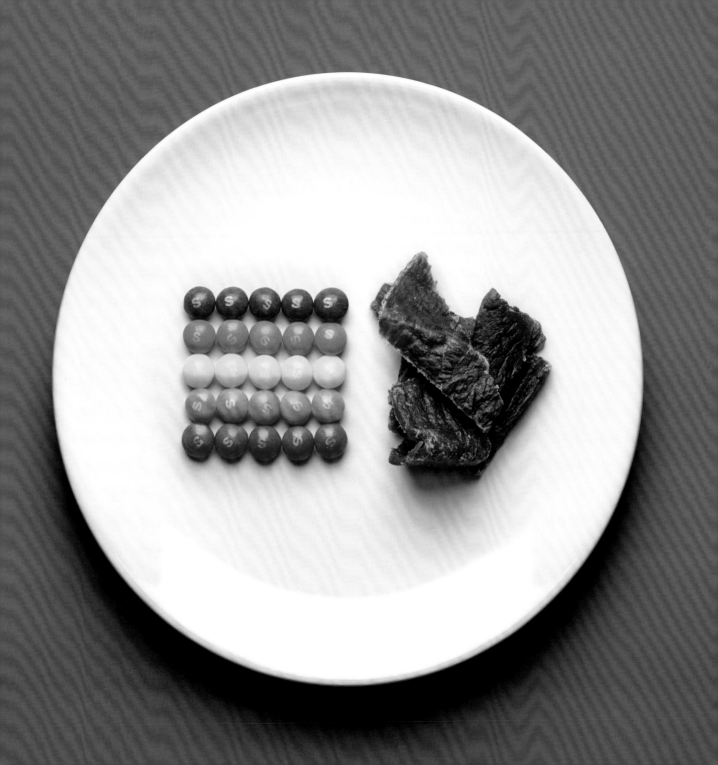

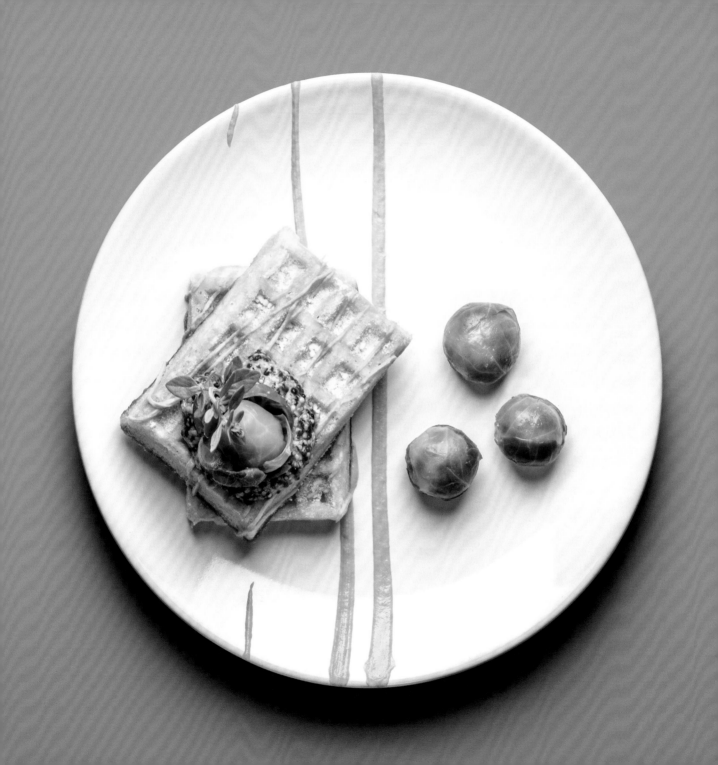

WAFFLES WITH MUSTARD AND BRUSSELS SPROUTS

Michele, Johnstown, Pennsylvania, USA

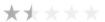

If you love Brussels sprouts, you might be able to appreciate this as a slightly offbeat waffle topping. If not, it's future vomit.

INGREDIENTS

1 egg

1 cup all-purpose flour

2 teaspoons sugar

¼ teaspoon vanilla extract

Pinch of salt

¾ cup / 180 ml milk

¼ cup / 60 ml sunflower oil

4 Brussels sprouts

1 tablespoon Dijon mustard

1 tablespoon mustard

METHOD

Heat up the waffle iron.

Beat the egg until light and fluffy.

Add the flour, sugar, vanilla extract, salt, milk, and oil and beat well.

Pour the mixture into the waffle iron (this recipe makes two waffles)

Cook until golden brown and crispy (4–5 minutes).

While you are cooking the waffles, bring a pot of water to a boil.

Add the Brussels sprouts and cook for 5–10 minutes until tender.

Remove the pot from the heat and drain.

Serve the waffles on a plate with the mustard and Brussels sprouts on top.

SERVES 1

MASHED POTATO
WITH CARAMEL SAUCE

Thalia, Johannesburg, South Africa

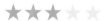

*Not quite as tasty as mashed potato without caramel sauce
or caramel sauce without mashed potato, but still strangely more-ish.*

SAUCE

1 cup brown sugar

3 tablespoons water

4 tablespoons butter

½ cup / 120 ml double cream

POTATOES

1 teaspoon salt

2 medium potatoes

1 tablespoon butter

¼ cup / 60 ml milk

METHOD

Make the caramel sauce first by putting the sugar and water in a large pan over low-medium heat. Stir until all the sugar has dissolved. Turn up the heat until it boils, stirring all the while. After a few minutes, remove the pan from the heat and stir in the butter and cream. Leave the sauce to cool a little while you make the potatoes.

Boil a pot of water and add the salt.

Peel the potatoes and cut them into quarters.

Boil the potatoes for about 15 minutes.

Drain.

Add the butter and milk and mash until smooth.

Add salt to taste.

Serve on a plate, pour the sauce on top, and enjoy.

SERVES 1

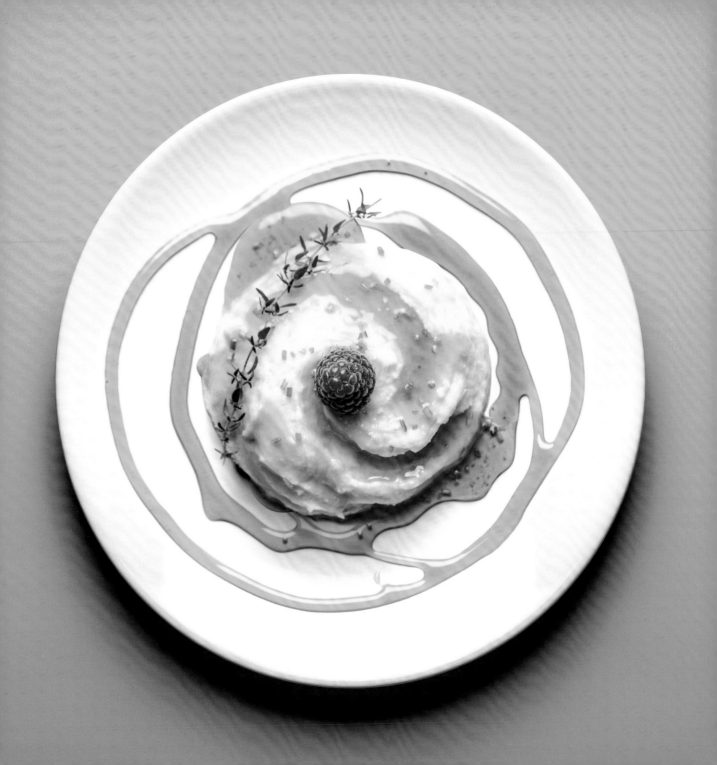

BUTTERED WATERMELON

Sarah, Toronto, Canada

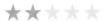

*The butter takes the delicate freshness of the watermelon to new heights . . .
and then pushes it off them, completely annihilating any trace of it.*

INGREDIENTS

¼ seedless watermelon

⅓ pound / 150 g butter

METHOD

Cut the watermelon into slices.

Remove the rind.

Cut the slices into pretentious, bite-size squares and spread
evenly with a generous layer of butter on top.

———————

SERVES 1

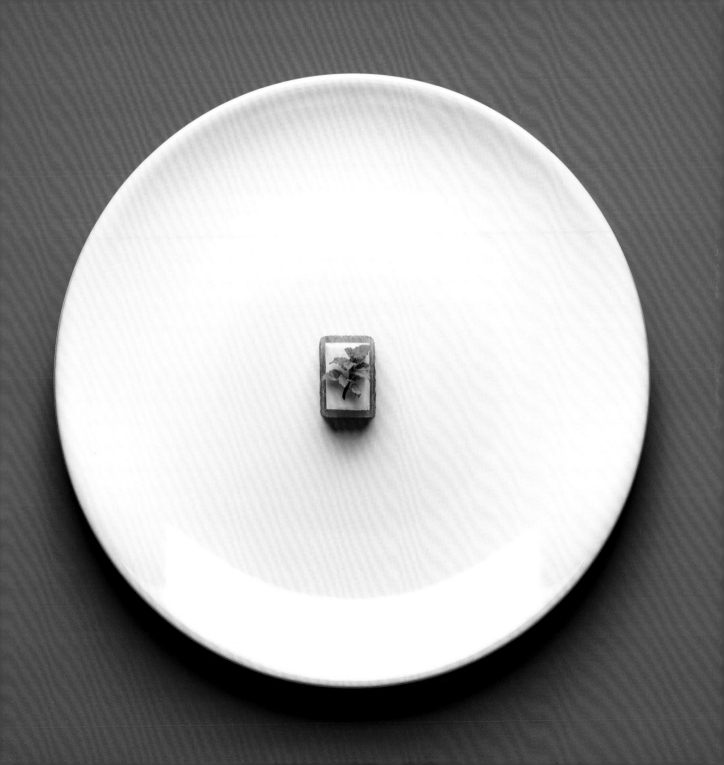

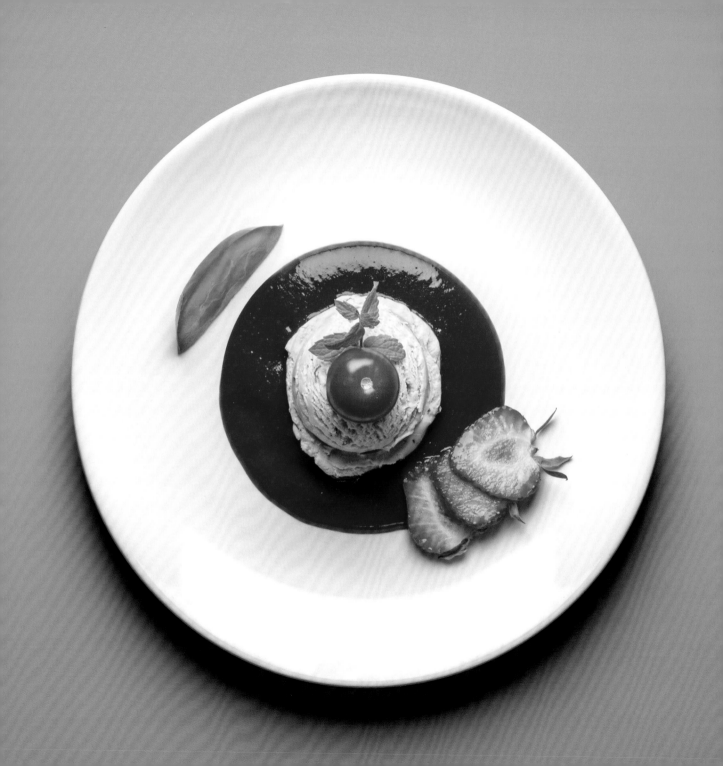

STRAWBERRY ICE CREAM AND KETCHUP

Remy, Washington DC, USA

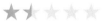

Ketchup is a rather unwelcome element. Kind of like when you put on your shoe without realizing there's a cockroach inside.

INGREDIENTS

Ketchup

Strawberry ice cream

METHOD

Put some ketchup on a scoop of strawberry ice cream.

————————————

SERVES 1

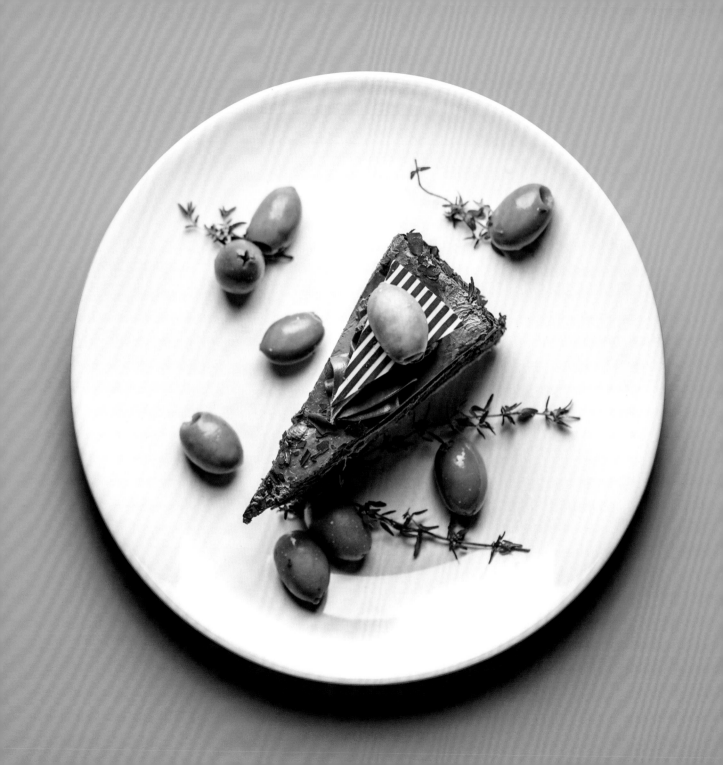

CHOC-OLIVE CAKE

Angela, Catalão, Goiás, Brazil

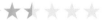

The perfect birthday cake for your enemies.

INGREDIENTS

½ cup / 120 g butter

1 cup milk

3 ounces / 90 g of cocoa

3 eggs

1 pound 2 ounces / 500 g white sugar

1 pound 2 ounces / 500 g
all-purpose flour

3 teaspoons baking powder

1 teaspoon vanilla extract

4 ounces / 120 g pitted green
olives, roughly chopped

ICING

1 pound 14 ounces / 400 g
confectioners' sugar

2 tablespoons boiling water

4 tablespoons cocoa powder

6 tablespoons butter

20 pitted green olives

METHOD

Preheat the oven to 350°F / 180°C.

Melt the butter and milk in a saucepan, then add the cocoa and bring the mixture to a boil stirring constantly to avoid lumps.

Remove the saucepan from the heat and leave to cool.

Beat the eggs and sugar in a bowl until the mixture becomes a creamy color.

Add the cocoa mixture from the saucepan along with the flour, baking powder, and vanilla extract to the egg mixture and beat for 1 minute. Stir in the chopped olives.

Bake for 30 minutes. Remove the pans from the oven and the cakes from the pans and then leave them to cool.

Begin making the icing by sifting the sugar into a bowl. Add the water to the cocoa powder to make a thick paste. Beat the paste, butter, and sugar together.

Frost one of the cooled cakes then place the other cake on top. Cover the top and sides of the cake with the rest of the icing. Use the green olives as decoration.

SERVES 1 . . . TWELVE TIMES OVER.

SPONGE

Melanie, Salisbury, Wiltshire, England

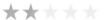

The flavor is a bit like the Loch Ness Monster. Or your left sock.
No matter how long or hard you search, you still can't seem to find it.

INGREDIENTS

1 sponge

1 tablespoon water

1 drop liquid soap

1 bowl lukewarm water,
for dipping

METHOD

Place the sponge on the plate.

Beat the drop of soap with the tablespoon of water until it has the appearance of whipped cream.

Arrange the beaten soap in a swirl on top of the sponge.

Serve with the bowl of water.

Dip the sponge in a bowl of water and chew on it.

_____

SERVES 0—PLEASE DON'T TRY THIS AT HOME. IN THE SHOWER, THE BATH, THE KITCHEN, OR ANYWHERE FOR THAT MATTER.

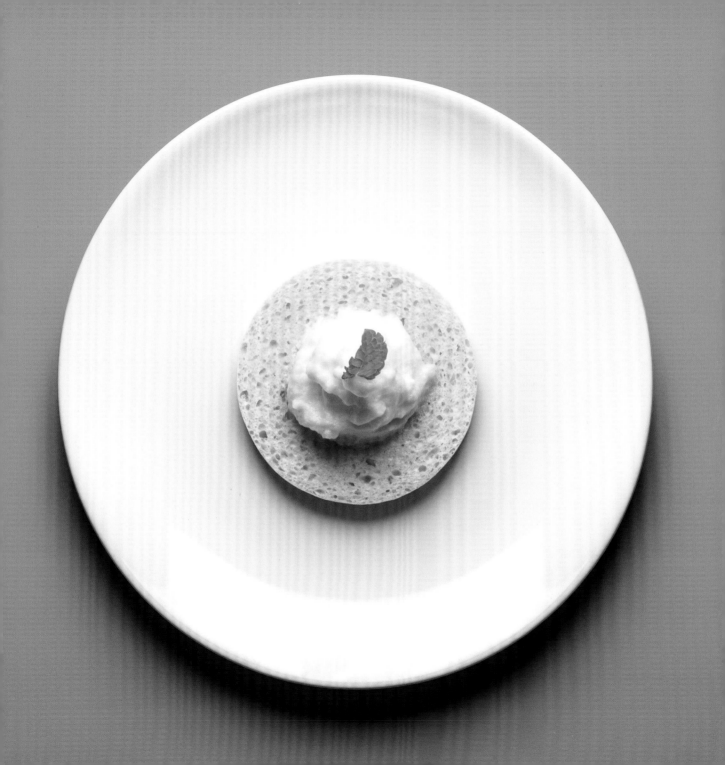

SPONGE

MELANIE, SALISBURY, WILTSHIRE, ENGLAND

I don't even really know how I got the idea to eat it. I was about six months pregnant and sitting in a (quite important and tense) work meeting, when suddenly I had an overwhelming urge to chew on a sponge. Not to eat it, as such, but just to chew it. The urge didn't go away for the rest of that day and I actually was worried it could have been a sign of a deficiency—the midwife recommended some blood tests to be sure, but there was nothing wrong—it was just a very weird pregnancy craving!

I had it every evening, in the bath. It was the highlight of my day! It got so bad though that at eight months pregnant I went away for three nights on a work trip and took my bath sponge with me—on the first night I WAS CHEWING ON IT IN THE SHOWER AND REALIZED IT WAS NEARLY FALLING APART AND NEEDED REPLACING, BUT I WASN'T GOING TO BE ABLE TO GET TO A SHOP UNTIL THE END OF THE WORK TRIP—I WAS SO STRESSED OUT BY IT! That's when I realized the difference between a real pregnancy craving and a 'normal' desire to eat something because you're pregnant and your body feels weird.

For a few days after my son was born it still tasted good, but then it was suddenly repulsive. I guess it must have been hormonal.

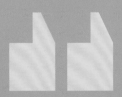

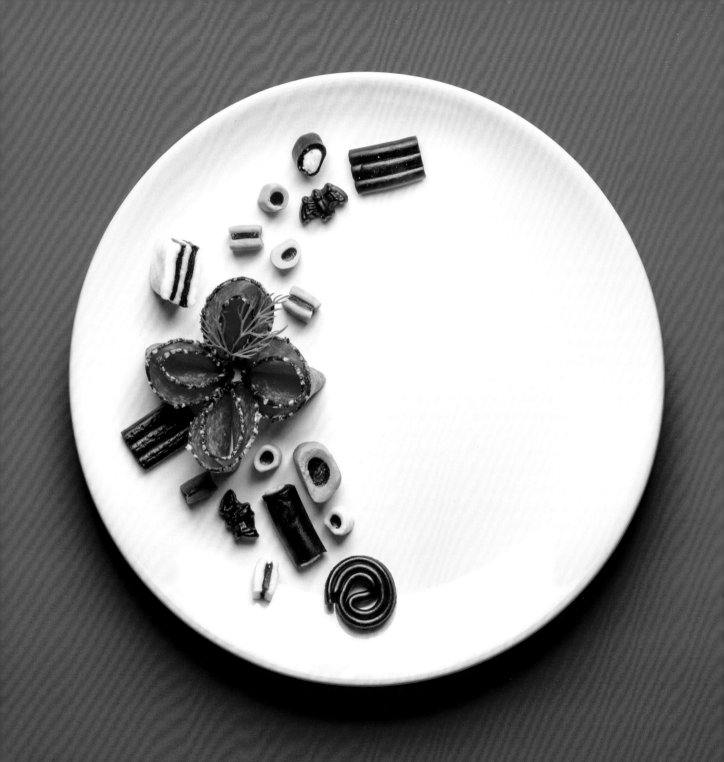

LICORICE AND SALAMI

Debbie, Athens, Greece

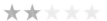

*Flavors that can tolerate each other, but just barely.
Like your family over the holiday season.*

INGREDIENTS

2–6 slices of salami

15–20 pieces of licorice

METHOD

Make salami flowers by folding the salami and securing it in place with a toothpick.

Arrange the licorice pieces on a plate.

Eat together.

SERVES 1

BRUSSELS SPROUT BLANCMANGE

Laura, Bridgend, South Wales, Wales

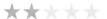

At least the pudding kills the taste of the Brussels sprouts somewhat.

INGREDIENTS

¼ teaspoon plain gelatin

2 teaspoons cold water

4 Brussels sprouts

Green food coloring

½ cup / 120 ml milk

¾ tablespoon cornstarch

1 tablespoon sugar

¼ teaspoon vanilla extract

METHOD

Soften the gelatin in the cold water and set aside.

Bring a pot of water to a boil and cook the Brussels sprouts until tender. This should take 5–10 minutes.

Remove the pot from the heat and drain, then rinse the sprouts under cold water to cool and pat dry.

Carefully remove the leaves from one of the Brussels sprouts. Keep the five best leaves for the top of the pudding and reserve the rest.

Add a little green food coloring to the gelatin, then pour half into the bottom of a mold.

Arrange your five Brussels sprout leaves carefully in an attractive pattern. Pour the rest of the gelatin in and leave to chill for about an hour or until set.

Mix half the milk with the cornstarch and sugar in a bowl.

Bring the other half of the milk to a boil with the reserved leaves of the Brussels sprout in it for extra flavor.

Strain the liquid to remove the leaves.

(recipe continues)

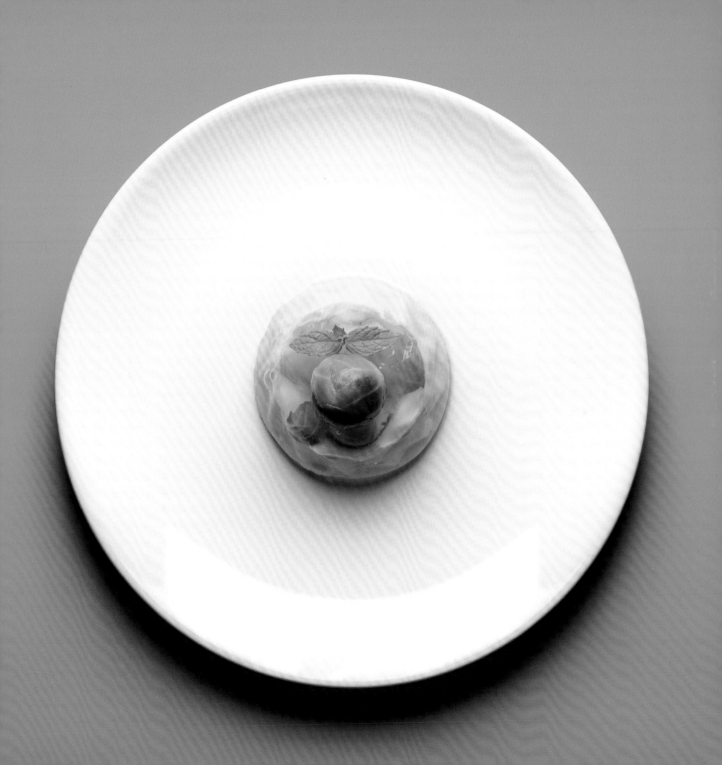

Slowly add the hot milk to the cold milk mixture, a little at a time, stirring constantly.

Cook on low heat for about 15 minutes stirring constantly.

Remove from the heat and add the vanilla extract.

Pour into the mold on top of the gelatin and chill overnight.

Remove from the mold and place one of the cooked Brussels sprouts on top.

Pull apart the leaves somewhat to create the appearance of a flower.

Serve.

SERVES 1

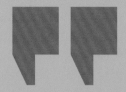

I THOUGHT THAT BRUSSELS SPROUTS AND BLANCMANGE TOGETHER WAS ABSOLUTELY AMAZING. I HAD IT AT LEAST ONCE A DAY. MY LITTLE ONE NOW HAS THE NICKNAME OF SPROUT.

BRUSSELS SPROUT BLANCMANGE

LAURA, BRIDGEND, SOUTH WALES, WALES

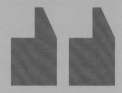

ORANGE SLICES
WITH TOMATO SAUCE GLAZE

Lindsay, Johannesburg, South Africa

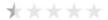

*The true evil in this dish is that it catches you unaware.
Who doesn't like oranges? Who doesn't like ketchup?
What harm could there be in putting them together? Why have I lost the will to live?*

INGREDIENTS

1 orange

Ketchup

*2 teaspoons orange zest,
for garnish*

METHOD

Cut the orange in half, then cut each half into six equal-size wedges.

Serve arranged on a plate covered in ketchup.

Sprinkle the orange zest on top as garnish.

SERVES 1

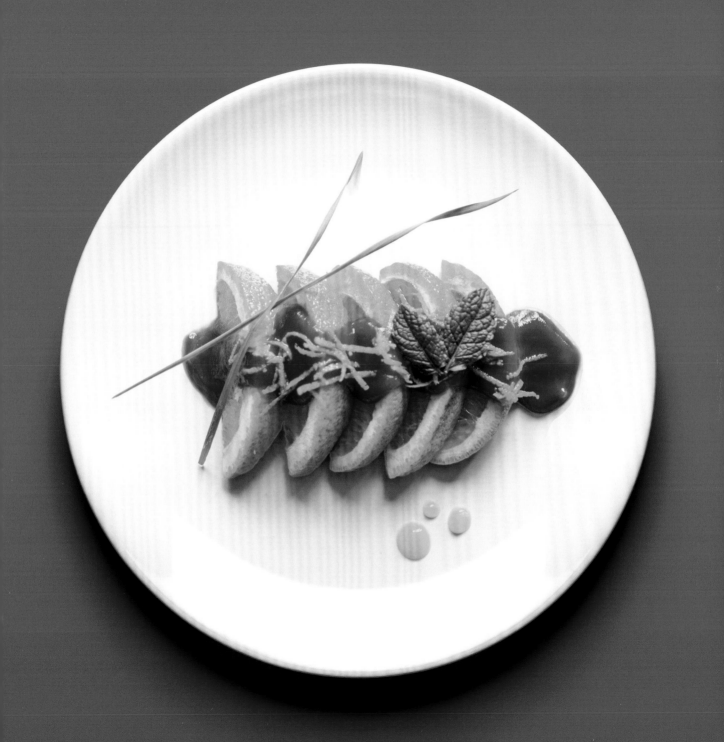

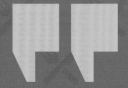

ORANGE SLICES WITH TOMATO SAUCE GLAZE

LINDSAY, JOHANNESBURG, SOUTH AFRICA

I had been obsessed with oranges since the start of my pregnancy, so when I invited my family over for dinner there was no question that oranges would be part of the menu. Orange sorbet, beautifully served in hollowed out orange peel "bowls" took my fancy. While carefully scraping the orange segments out of the skin I would pop a piece into my mouth every now and then.

Working steadily through the oranges, I suddenly felt that their natural flavor could be improved somehow. After some trial and error with salt, pepper, and sugar, on a whim I decided to try tomato sauce. It was a winner! Confident that I had discovered a sensational combo, that evening I URGED MY GUESTS TO TRY IT . . . THEY STILL ACCUSE ME OF TRYING TO POISON THEM TO THIS DAY.

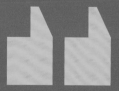

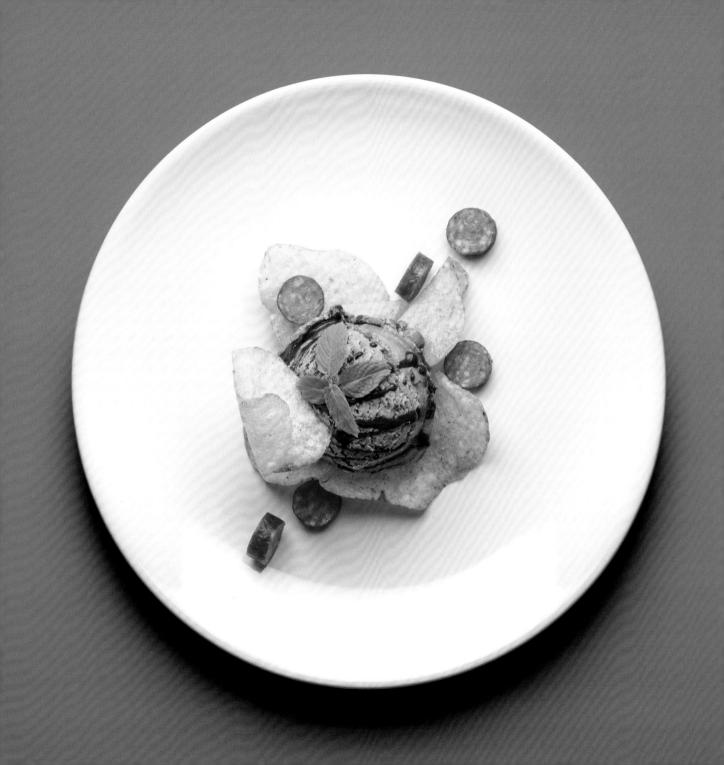

ICE CREAM, CHIPS, AND BEEF STICKS

Sandy, New York, USA

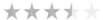

The chips give it a salty crunch. The ice cream makes a cool, creamy base.
The beef sticks are a bit overpowering, but they aren't necessarily a flavor clash.
It's one of those things that sounds like it shouldn't work, but it does.
Like a duck-billed platypus.

INGREDIENTS

Handful of plain salted potato chips

1 scoop of chocolate ice cream

½ beef stick, sliced

METHOD

Make a bed of chips on the plate, reserving one.

Place the scoop of ice cream on top.

Stick the remaining chip into the ice cream like a wafer.

Sprinkle the dish with beef stick slices.

Serve.

SERVES 1

HOT DOG AND PICKLE SMOOTHIE

Shivawn, Chicago, USA

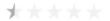

*It takes a moment before you feel it, but then it hits you right
in the stomach and you find yourself curled up on the floor whimpering.
In short, if you don't have testicles, this is your opportunity
to find out what it is like to be kicked in them.*

INGREDIENTS

1 hot dog bun

1 large pickle, sliced

1 hot dog, roughly chopped, with 2
neat slices reserved for garnish

Mustard

Relish

4 ice cubes

2 shots espresso

½ cup / 120 ml milk

4 tablespoons caramel sauce

Handful of whole
coffee beans, for garnish

4 slices of cornichon, for garnish

METHOD

In a food processor, blend the hot dog bun until
it is smoothly crumbed.

Reserve some pickle and hot dog slices for garnish

Add the rest of the nongarnish ingredients and blend well.

Pour into a glass, add garnish, and enjoy.

SERVES 1

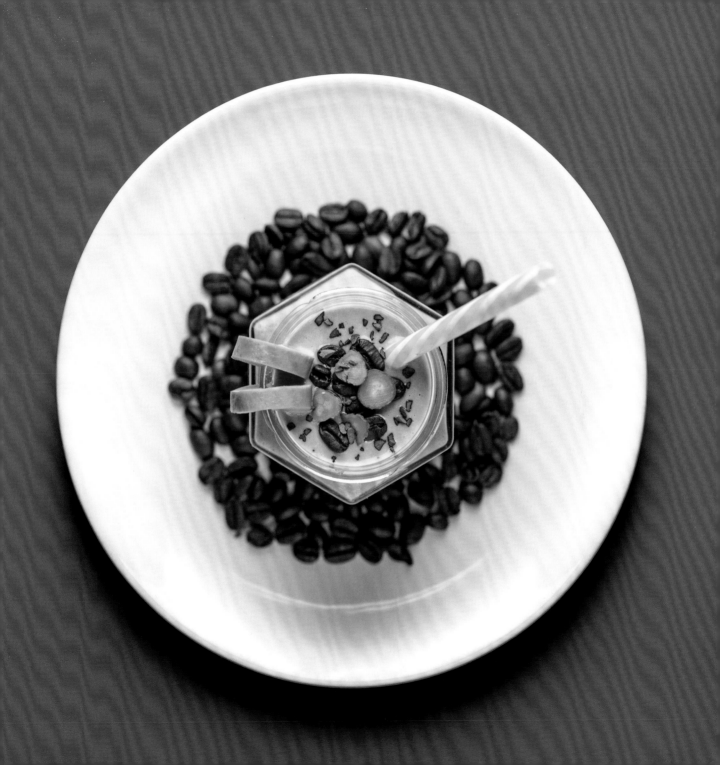

HOT DOG AND PICKLE SMOOTHIE

SHIVAWN, CHICAGO, USA

I started eating it before I even took a pregnancy test. THE FIRST TIME I TRIED IT MY HUSBAND LOOKED AT ME AND SAID, "YEAH, YOU'RE PREGNANT." When I first tasted it, I thought, "This is a little weird, but good!" . . . the tanginess of the mustard and relish mixing with the salty pickle and sweet coffee drink, I was instantly hooked. I was craving sweet/salty/tangy and it hit the spot. Guess you could say it's my version of pickles and ice cream . . . with a hot dog to help fill me up.

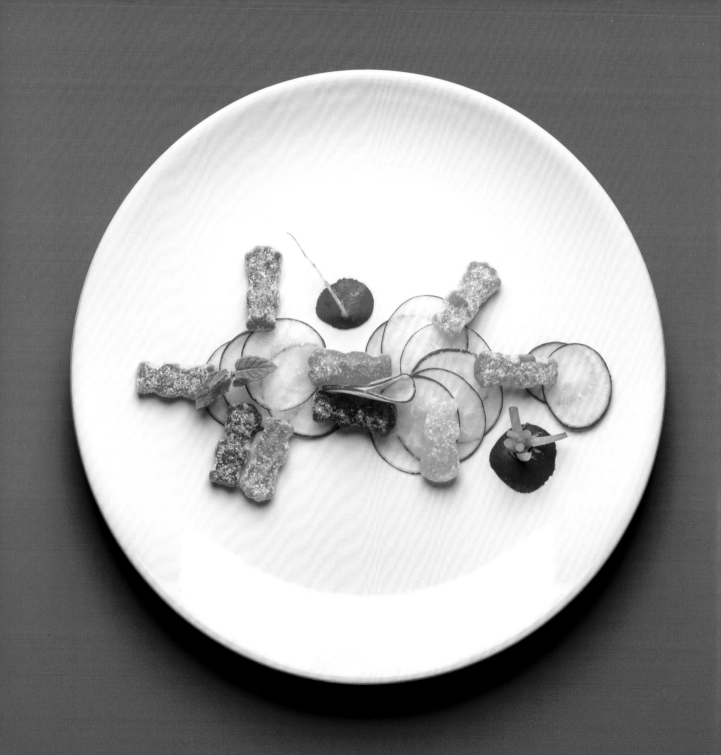

SOUR RADISH PATCH

Shannon, Pepin, Wisconsin, USA

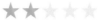

The radishes add a pleasant crunch but an unpleasant vegetable-y aftertaste. You can almost hear the Sour Patch Kids saying "Moooom, do we have to?"

INGREDIENTS

2 radishes

8–15 Sour Patch Kids / sour candy

METHOD

Wash the radishes well.

Slice them thinly, about 1/10 inch / 3 mm thick.

Place the sour candy on top.

When eating, wrap each candy in a slice or two of radish like you are giving each Sour Patch Kid a blanket and tucking it in.

SERVES 1

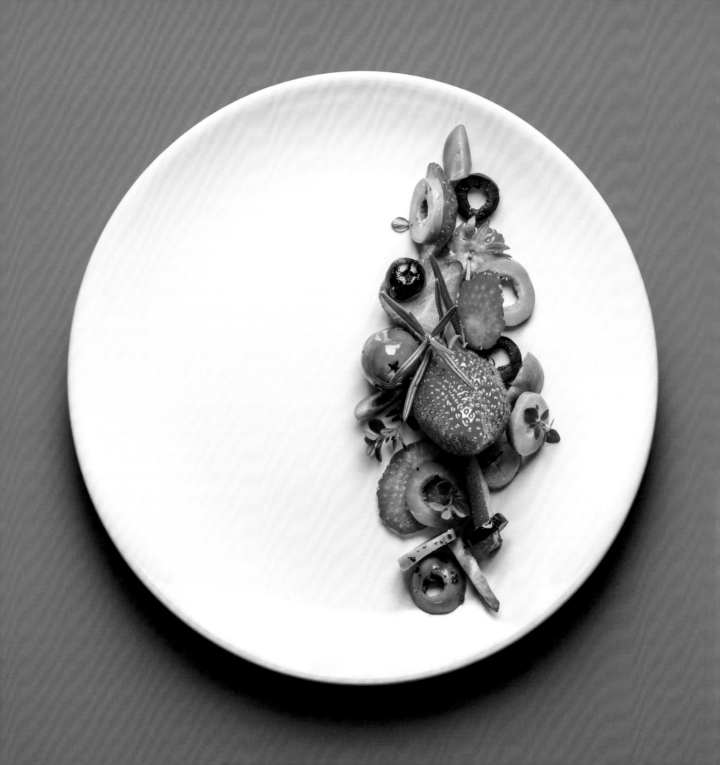

OLIVES AND STRAWBERRY SALAD

Amanda, São Paulo, Brazil

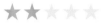

Nope nope nope nope nope nope nope nope nope nope

INGREDIENTS

2 ounces / 55 g strawberries

2 ounces / 55 g pitted green olives

METHOD

Wash the strawberries and slice.

Put them in a bowl, add the olives, and toss until they are mixed well.

Serve.

Question your life choices.

SERVES 1

BANANAS WITH HOT DOG CHILI

Bella, Cleveland, Ohio, USA

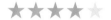

*Your alarm clock doesn't go off and you are late for work. On a day
there is a meeting with your boss. For your yearly review. It goes badly.
Very badly. "Pack-your-stuff-and-be-out-by-the-end-of-the-day" badly. On the way
out, you accidentally step in a giant mud puddle ruining your favorite shoes . . .
just as a passing bird relieves itself on your head. When you finally get home,
your key breaks off in the door. Four hours later, after emptying the contents of your
wallet into the locksmith's pocket, you have finally gained entry to your house. It is late at night
before you realize that today was actually your birthday. But that's OK.
Nobody else remembered either. You go to the fridge and all you have left
is a banana and some leftover hot dog chili. You eat them
and that night you go to sleep happy, knowing the world really
is a wonderful place.*

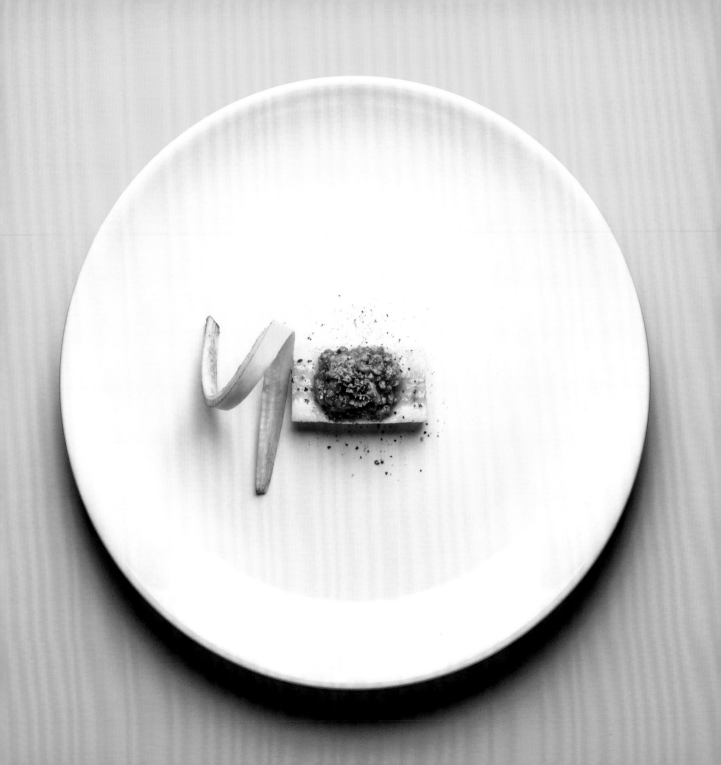

INGREDIENTS

½ onion, finely chopped

2 tablespoons oil

1 clove of garlic

5 ounces / 150 g ground beef

Salt

Pepper

Pinch of chili powder

1 teaspoon paprika

¼ (14-ounce / 400-ml) can tomato puree

1 tablespoon ketchup

1 teaspoon sugar

2 bananas

Parsley, for garnish

METHOD

Fry the onion in the oil over medium heat until translucent.

Add the garlic and ground beef.

Make sure to continue breaking up the ground beef while it cooks so that it has a fine consistency.

Add the salt, pepper, chili powder, and paprika to the ground beef mixture.

Pour in the tomato puree and add the ketchup and sugar.

Simmer for 15 minutes on low heat.

Peel the bananas and slice lengthwise, then into bite-size pieces about 1½ inches (4 cm) long.

Put a dollop of hot dog chili on top of each banana square.

Garnish with a little fresh parsley and enjoy.

SERVES 2—YOU ARE GOING TO WANT A SECOND HELPING

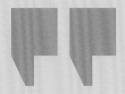

I GOT THE IDEA WHEN MY HUSBAND WAS EATING A BANANA WHILE I WAS EATING HOT DOG CHILI. I WAS SO HUNGRY IT SOUNDED AMAZING. WHEN I TRIED IT I THOUGHT IT WAS THE GREATEST THING EVER. MY HUSBAND JUST HAD A LOOK OF "YUCK" ON HIS FACE.

BANANAS WITH HOT DOG CHILE

BELLA, CLEVELAND, OHIO, USA

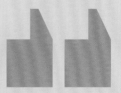

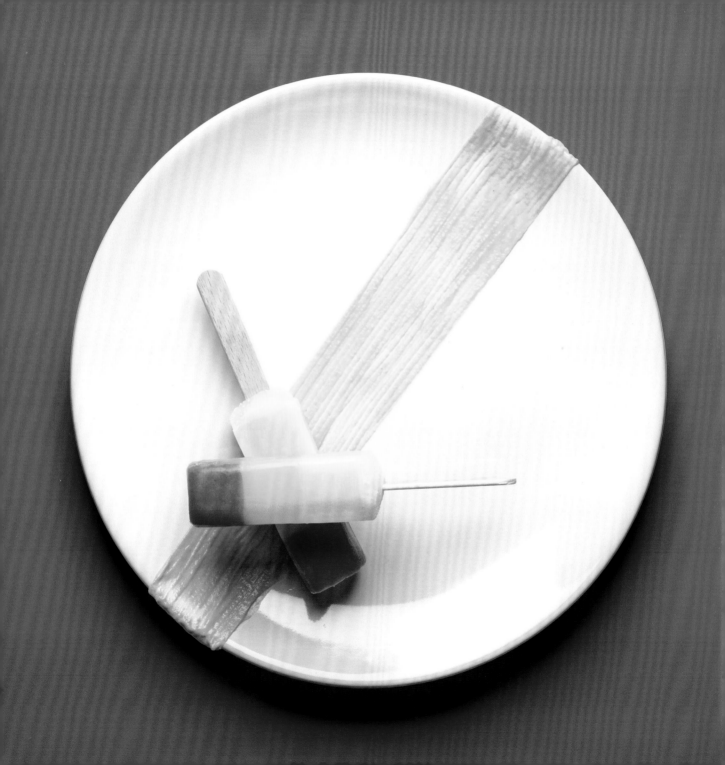

POPSICLES AND MUSTARD

Laura, Liverpool, England

....

★★✮★★

The effect on your tongue is to instantly form the word "Why?"

....

INGREDIENTS

2 tablespoons mustard

3 popsicles

METHOD

Make a stripe or bed of mustard on your plate.

Cut one popsicle into slices.

Arrange the popsicles and slices on the plate.

———————————

SERVES 1

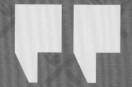

POPSICLES AND MUSTARD

LAURA, LIVERPOOL, ENGLAND

I WAS OBSESSED WITH MUSTARD WHILST PREGNANT BUT ALSO HAD NINE MONTHS OF MORNING/NOON/NIGHT SICKNESS SO I HAD TO EAT LOLLY ICES TO ENSURE I HAD SOME FLUID INTAKE. MY LITTLE GIRL WAS BORN WITH BLONDE HAIR, WHICH THEN TURNED A VIBRANT RED ON HER SECOND DAY—I BLAME THE MUSTARD.

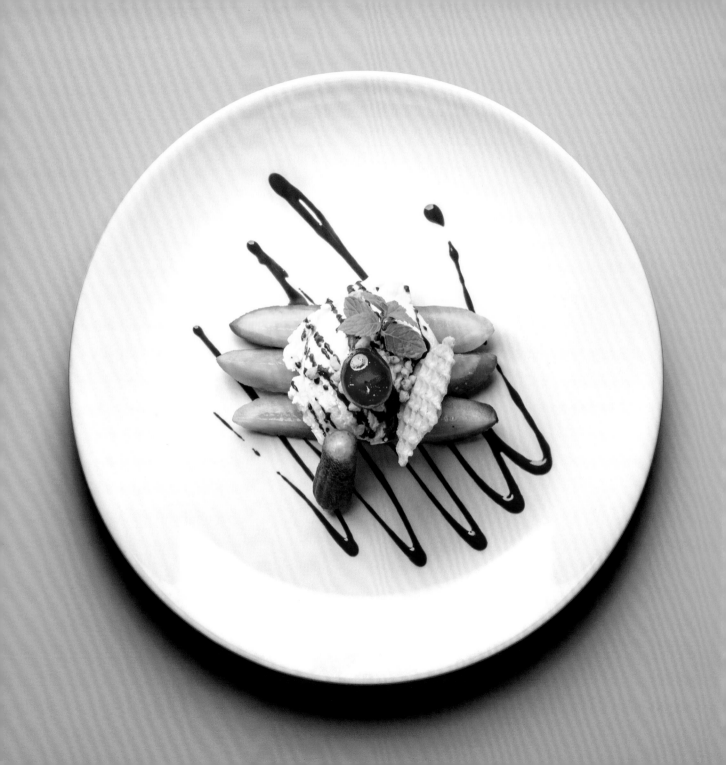

PICKLES AND ICE CREAM

Maria, Sturgis, Michigan, USA

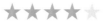

This is so delicious we actually took a pregnancy test just to make sure neither of us was pregnant. Even the one with a penis.

INGREDIENTS

3 dill pickle spears

1 scoop of vanilla ice cream

Chocolate sauce

1 cornichon, for "spoon"

1 Maraschino cherry, for garnish

METHOD

Place the pickle spears parallel to each other on the plate.

Put the scoop of ice cream on top so that it is riding the pickle-spear skis.

Dribble the chocolate sauce over the ice cream.

Add the cornichon to use as a spoon and put the cherry on top.

SERVES 1

THE COUNTDOWN:
TOP 10 BIGGEST CRAVINGS

When we started collecting and hoarding cravings like pregnancy-obsessed hamsters, patterns quickly began to emerge. We kept encountering the same foods over and over (times infinity) again. This is a list of pregnancy's biggest hits. The rock stars of cravings that all maternity wear shops should keep in the impulse-buy aisle.

10. FAST FOOD

The thing with fast food is that almost all nonpregnant people also have a burning desire to stuff it into their food-hole. But it can't be denied, we did come across a lot of McDonalds, KFC, and Burger King cravings. Since fast food is an excellent source of pretty much nothing except calories, it seems most likely that it is just a magnification of a normal craving because people are now eating for two.

9. WATERMELON

"Let's have watermelon for dinner!" said ~~no one ever.~~ a lot of pregnant women. Alone or in a whacky combination, watermelon is the summer fruit everyone forgot about until they were impregnated. And there is good reason it keeps making a comeback on pregnant women's shopping lists: watermelon is the Superman of maternity foods. Although it is mostly water, it is water absolutely drenched in vitamins A, B$_6$, and C, lycopene, antioxidants, and amino acids. "Can water *really* be drenched in things?" you say. Yes. Now stop asking irrelevant questions and let's get back to the wondermelon. Because of its high water and nutrient content, it can help with heartburn, swelling, and morning sickness—you know, all those things soon-to-be-moms keep mentioning are a teeny weeny bit uncomfortable. So let's hear it for the watermelon. Defeater of Morning Sickness, Queen of Nutrients, Destroyer of Heartburn, Wateriest of Melons.

8. MUSTARD

Slathered on muffins or popsicles, together with sardines and coffee, or even eaten directly out of the jar, mustard just kept popping up everywhere. It was like one of those new trends that you just can't believe people are doing. And then you can't believe how many people are doing it. Then, suddenly you seem to be the only one not doing it. And just like with all of those regrettable perms, mullets, awkward facial hair, and visible G-strings, people tend to look back on that period of their lives and ask themselves, "What the hell was I thinking?" It turns out that pregnant women's bodies are probably thinking "selenium." Mustard is an excellent source of this trace element, which is very important for the nervous and immune system of the fetus. Low selenium levels are also linked to miscarriage or low birth weight. It's even good for men's fertility, too. So give the mustard a high five and keep your judge-y eyes to yourself if you happen to see a pregnant woman drowning her popsicle in mustard.

7. ICE

We heard stories of women eating so much ice they chipped their teeth. And how many had freezers packed full of nothing but ice and partners who were driven to insanity by the incessant crunching. Another thing many of them had was anemia. It appears ice soothes inflammation in the mouth—one of the symptoms of anemia. So if you find yourself throwing your pizza and ice cream away to make space for ice, be sure to make an appointment at the doctor. And hey . . . if you aren't going to eat that pizza . . .

6. SPICY THINGS

Whether it be Flamin' Hot Cheetos, hot peppers, hot sauce, hot sauce, hot sauce, or hot sauce, there is a good chance it has a rabid fan club of pregnant women. It may be because hot foods make you sweat, which actually helps you keep cool. It may be because pregnancy turns your taste buds into crazy little aliens. Whatever the reason, a bottle of hot sauce in the bag when there wasn't one before is a good reason to suspect a baby in a belly where there wasn't one before.

5. DIRT AND OTHER NONFOOD CRAVINGS

Dirt, bricks, laundry detergent, soap, toothpaste, nail polish, matches, and sponges are just some of the items that make it onto the Weird Yet Weirdly Common Pregnancy Cravings list. Nonfood cravings, or pica, are way more prevalent in pregnancy than most people are aware of. And more so in developing countries. In Denmark 1 in 10,000 women admitted to eating dirt or clay when they were pregnant. But in Kenya, 1 in 2 did. That's right. Half. And just like with ice, nonfood cravings are often (but not always) related to anemia or other deficiencies. The moral of the story is if you are craving anything unusual, talk to your doctor about it. The other moral of the story is that pregnancy most definitely isn't for sissies.

4. PEANUT BUTTER

Everyone knows good ol' peanut butter and jelly. But what about peanut butter and onions? Or peanut butter with scrambled eggs? Or peanut butter with hot dogs? All these lesser-known PB&s have been eaten—and adored—by pregnant women. There was a time in the early 2000s that doctors were advising women not to eat peanuts when they were expecting, to avoid nut allergies in their children. But times have changed, as times often do. And the latest, most up-to-datest advice seems to be that eating peanuts and peanut butter might actually lessen the possibility of allergic reactions. Plus peanut butter is packed with some good stuff for mother and baby, like folate and antioxidants. Which means if you are pregnant and craving peanut butter, feel free to indulge and create your own weird and wonderful PB& combination.

3. ANYTHING SOUR

It is possible that we hold the dubious distinction of having heard the word "pickle" more than anyone else on the planet. But we also discovered that while women from the United States are likely to grab a pickle in times of pregnancy, women in Poland make a beeline for the pickled herring. Women in Germany stock up on sauerkraut and women in the United Kingdom often reach for a pack of salt and vinegar chips. Because it turns out many pregnant women LOVE sour things. It wasn't the pickle after all, it was the pickling! Vinegar was what all these women were after. Having exposed the pickle for the shameless credit-stealing vegetable that it is, we patted ourselves on the back for our amazing detective work, put our pipes in our mouths and returned to Baker Street. But not before exposing a few more culprits along the way (lemon and sour candy to be specific). The current theory is that craving sour things makes pregnant women eat a wider variety of foods and therefore a more balanced diet. Elementary, my dear Watson.

2. CHOCOLATE

Maybe it is because chocolate is a great source of magnesium. Maybe it is because chocolate is the most amazing thing in the world. Whatever the reason, one in seven of the recipes in this book contain chocolate in some form. It is safe to say chocolate and pregnancy go together like chocolate and Valentine's Day. Or chocolate and breakups. Or chocolate and Halloween. Or chocolate and Easter. Or chocolate at the movies. Or chocolate at midnight, unwrapped with the utmost stealth so you don't have to share. In fact, it is quite hard to find something that chocolate *doesn't* go with. Very hard but not impossible (see page 169, Shrimp with White Chocolate)

1. ICE CREAM WITH . . .

The cliché is true. Pregnant women are keeping the ice cream industry afloat. And Pickles and Ice Cream is definitely a thing. There is also an impressive degree of creativity in their ice cream toppings. Popcorn, hot sauce, ketchup, French fries, chicken, beef sticks, and steak are just a few of the combinations we came across. We are relatively confident that, if you can eat it, a pregnant woman somewhere has put it on ice cream.

SOURCES

Watermelon

www.livescience.com/46019-watermelon-nutrition.html

www.fitpregnancy.com/nutrition/prenatal-nutrition/watermelon-wonders?utm_source=
Fit%20Pregnancy_FACEBOOK_Nutrition&utm_medium=Evergreen&utm_campaign=Editorial%2
Content_20160605153000_484130914

Mustard

www.ncbi.nlm.nih.gov/pubmed/25175508

Ice

health.howstuffworks.com/wellness/food-nutrition/facts/why-does-anemia-make-people-want-
to-crunch-on-ice-1.htm

www.sheknows.com/food-and-recipes/articles/985411/foods-craved-by-pregnant-women

Spicy Things

www.sheknows.com/food-and-recipes/articles/985411/foods-craved-by-pregnant-women

Dirt and Other Nonfood Cravings

theweek.com/articles/485983/why-pregnant-women-eat-dirt

Peanut Butter

www.babycenter.com/404_is-it-safe-to-eat-peanut-butter-during-pregnancy_10315711.bc

Anything Sour

www.babble.com/pregnancy/science-why-pregnancy-food-cravings/

LABOR

THE MOMS

First and foremost we would like to thank all the women who opened up to us about their cravings and made this book possible. Their infinite patience with all our annoying questions only goes to prove what awesome moms they are. When we began this project, we had no idea how many wonderful, funny, and interesting people we would meet during the process. This book is dedicated to all of you. And moms with crazy cravings everywhere.

THE MIDWIVES

We would also like to thank the people without whom the delivery of this book would have been a lot more painful.

Sue Lopes for her frosting fierceness.

Our neighbors and BFFs Maria Cardoso and Diogo Alves for that indispensable pan, emergency supplies, and moral support.

Christian Asmar and Gabriel Pastor Hernandez for the mixer, the pickling advice, and patience with our whining.

Vicky's mom for being there on the day it all started and giving a few unhelpful but mostly very helpful suggestions.

Vicky's dad for trying the chalk recipe with us and his eloquent review of "Yuk."

Juarez's mom and dad for having him.

Tammy for her support, advice, and connections.

Jenya, Maks, and Axel for the translations of recipe submissions we couldn't understand.

Jennifer Kasius, our ever-helpful editor, and Running Press, our publishers.

All the blogs and websites that posted our project and the people who wrote to us about it— we were blown away by all the positive feedback.